MATHEMATICAL IDEAS
IN BIOLOGY

MATHEMATICAL IDEAS IN BIOLOGY

J. MAYNARD SMITH

Dean of the School of Biological Sciences
University of Sussex

CAMBRIDGE
AT THE UNIVERSITY PRESS
1968

Published by the Syndics of the Cambridge University Press
Bentley House, 200 Euston Road, London, N.W. 1
American Branch: 32 East 57th Street, New York, N.Y. 10022

Library of Congress Catalogue Card Number: 68–25088

Standard Book Number: 521 07335 9 cloth bound
                      521 09550 6 paperback

Printed in Great Britain
at the University Printing House, Cambridge
(Brooke Crutchley, University Printer)

CONTENTS

Appendices

To the memory of J. B. S. Haldane

INTRODUCTION

My aim in this book has been to show that mathematical reasoning is sometimes illuminating in biology.

It is widely assumed—particularly by statisticians—that the only branch of mathematics necessary for a biologist is statistics. I do not share this view. Statistics is necessary to biologists, because no two organisms are identical. But I have the feeling that statistics, and particularly that branch of it which deals with significance tests, has been over-sold. In any case, there are a number of admirable text books of statistics intended for biologists, and consequently I have nothing to add here.

In contrast, I am concerned in this book with those branches of mathematics—primarily differential equations, recurrence relations and probability theory—which can be used to describe biological processes. The advantage which biologists would gain from a knowledge of these subjects has been largely ignored. The reason for this neglect is I think as follows. It is comparatively easy to learn the calculus, and there are a number of excellent books from which it can be learnt. But unfortunately it is very difficult to turn biological problems into differential equations. Consequently few biologists bother to learn the calculus, since they cannot see what they would do with it if they knew it. It is this problem of the translation of biological problems into mathematical terms which is my main topic.

The book has been written primarily for biologists, who increasingly will need to read papers containing mathematical reasoning, and who will occasionally need to use mathematics in their own work. Indeed if a biologist can learn enough mathematics to know when the problem he is working on could usefully be discussed with a mathematical colleague, that alone will be worth considerable effort. Consequently I have approached mathematics in the spirit of one trying to teach French to a prospective visitor to Paris, and not to one about to sit an examination in French grammar. What matters is that you should start using mathematics as a language, not that you should never make a mistake.

However I hope that the book will be of some interest to mathematicians, particularly to those who have to teach mathematics to biologists, and to those who are seeking fields for the application of mathematics in biology. Inevitably a mathematician will be irritated by this book, because I have solved particular problems instead of dealing with the general case, and I have used crude methods when elegant ones were possible. Nevertheless I may have done enough to show how one can start applying mathematics to biology.

Any attempt to apply mathematics to the world involves three stages. Suppose for example we want to use mathematics to study the behaviour of a weight suspended on a spring. First we use what we know about mechanics and about springs to write down an equation—usually a differential equation—describing the behaviour of the weight; in this case the appropriate equation is $d^2x/dt^2 + kx = 0$. We then temporarily forget about the real world, and use purely mathematical reasoning to 'solve' this equation; in this case, we find that $x = a\sin\sqrt{k}t$. Finally we return to the real world, and interpret this solution as meaning that the weight will oscillate harmonically with a period $2\pi/\sqrt{k}$.

In biology, the difficult stage is the first one. We rarely know enough about the laws governing the components of biological systems to be able to write down the appropriate equation with any confidence in the first place. If an equation can be written down, it is usually possible to find a mathematician who will solve it, and if this is impossible, solutions can be found by a computer. The interpretation stage does not often present any great difficulty.

Consequently, I have been more concerned in these pages to explain how equations can be written down than to describe how they can be solved. There are some areas of biology—notably in genetics—where the 'laws' are fairly well understood. In population genetics therefore there has been built up a structure of mathematical reasoning similar to that found in most branches of physics. But in most other areas there are no laws which can be used with the same confidence as that with which geneticists use Mendel's laws. In population genetics we know the way genes segregate in sexual reproduction, and we use this knowledge to predict how populations will evolve. In most areas of biology, we know as much or more about the behaviour of a whole system than we do about its parts, and we would like to be able to deduce the properties of the parts from the behaviour of the whole. There is usually no direct way of doing this. What we can do is to make plausible guesses about the properties of the parts, and then deduce how the system as a whole would behave if these guesses were true. By comparing our deductions with the known behaviour of the system we can see how adequate our original guesses were.

To give one example of this procedure, the physicist Leo Szilard produced a theory of ageing based on the assumption that ageing is due to the accumulation of recessive mutations in non-dividing cells. His theory predicted several consequences (e.g. that inbred animals should live longer than outbred ones) which are known not to be the case. The theory was therefore valuable in helping to disprove its original assumptions, although it must be admitted that its author did not see it in this light.

It follows that there really is some point in trying to formulate biological problems in mathematical language, even when we know too little to make the formulation precise. Another advantage of the attempt at mathematical formulation is that it helps to clarify which properties of the components of a system must be known if its behaviour is to be predicted; in other words, it tells us what we need to measure.

I have confined myself to strictly biological topics; fortunately, many of the same mathematical tools are useful in analysing other systems which, although not themselves biological, are of importance to some biologists—for example, the kinetics of chemical reactions, or the behaviour of electrical circuits. Within biology, I have tried to choose topics about which it is possible to say something illuminating with quite simple mathematical language.

In general, each chapter could be read by itself, and the chapters could be read in any order, although chapters 2 and 3 should be read in that order, and likewise chapters 4 and 5. Nevertheless, the same mathematical ideas recur in different contexts in different chapters, and I have tried to underline this when it happens. One of the major illuminations conferred by mathematics is to show the logical and structural similarities between systems which at first sight are quite different; for example, no control engineer could look at the Canadian game cycle, or for that matter at an economic cycle of boom and slump, without asking himself where the delay in the feedback loop occurs.

A major problem has been to decide how much mathematical knowledge to assume in my readers. As a starting point I have assumed a knowledge of elementary mathematics only. In particular, I assume the reader can solve quadratic equations, plot graphs of algebraic functions, and is familiar with the idea of differentiation and integration of functions such as $3x^2$ or $4x - 5x^5$. Where mathematical knowledge beyond this level is required, I have included a brief account in an appendix. These appendices cover a wide area (including circular functions, exponential and logarithmic functions, complex numbers, linear recurrence relations and linear differential equations) in a very few words. All the topics are dealt with in greater detail and with greater rigour in text books of mathematics for scientists. The appendices in this book are not intended to provide rigorous proofs of the various theorems stated. I shall be satisfied if I have said enough to show the reader what kind of thing is being said in these theorems, and to convince him that they are not wholly implausible. My advice to those meeting complex numbers, or the idea that $\sin \theta$ can be expressed as an infinite series, for the first time, is to operate with these ideas without bothering too much about proofs or justifications. Historically, people used these ideas quite happily for a long time before adequate definitions or proofs had been given. Once you have convinced yourself of the utility of the fact that

$$e^{i\theta} = \cos \theta + i \sin \theta,$$

you will soon convince yourself of its truth.

I have from time to time used numerical methods of solving equations in this book. I am convinced that to solve equations numerically is a good habit to acquire. It is also a good thing to learn that many equations cannot be solved analytically, but can easily be solved numerically. I remember that the first problem I met when I started work as an engineer required that I evaluate $\int x \tan x \, dx$. I spent most of a day trying to find an analytical solution before it occurred to me to plot a graph and add up the squares. An additional reason for encouraging people to use numerical methods is that such methods need no longer be laborious, since a computer will do the work. Of course analytical solutions are preferable. But a numerical solution of the actual problem may be preferable to an analytical solution of an over-simplified version of the problem.

Finally, I have included a number of examples at the end of each chapter. Biologists do not always appreciate that to learn mathematics requires practice just as much as learning to play the piano. It is my impression that the examples will prove to be rather difficult. But I am sure that time spent solving them will not be wasted, particularly because some of the examples illustrate points of biological as well as of mathematical interest.

1   SOME CONSEQUENCES OF SCALE

This chapter illustrates three topics: first, a method of thinking about the effects of size on the shape and performance of animals; second, the application of the laws of mechanics to animal locomotion; and third, the idea that animal structure can be thought of as optimising particular functions.

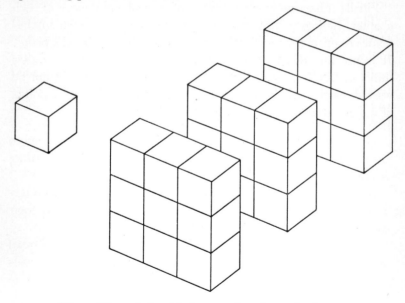

Fig. 1. The relationship between lengths and volumes.

A. The idea of dimension

Consider first the problem of scale. It is shown in fig. 1 that if two cubes are compared, one with edges three times as long as the other, the surface area of the larger cube is 9 times greater, and its volume is 27 times greater. This can be generalised in two stages:

(i) If two cubes have edges in the ratio $1:L$, their surface areas are in the ratio $1:L^2$, and their volumes in the ratio $1:L^3$.

(ii) If two shapes are geometrically similar, and if the distance between two points on one of them is to the distance between the two corresponding points on the other in the ratio $1:L$, then corresponding areas are in the ratio $1:L^2$, and corresponding volumes in the ratio $1:L^3$.

In what follows, we shall discuss sets of geometrically similar animals, differing only in size, and discuss how their performance of different tasks would vary. If animals differ in size but not in shape, then if the shape of one is known, any other can be described by a single representative length L—for example the total height, or the length of a particular bone.

The most familiar effect of scale on animals concerns the ability of their skeletons to support their weight. The argument is as follows:

(i) The ability of a bone to withstand a direct compression or tension load is proportional to its cross-sectional area, and hence to L^2. For example, an animal three times as high as another would have limbs able to withstand 9 times the weight.

(ii) The weight to be supported by the limbs is proportional to the volume, and hence to L^3. For example, an animal three times as high would weigh 27 times as much.

(iii) It follows that if land animals increased in size indefinitely without change of shape, their skeletons could not support their weight.

In fact, larger mammals are not geometrically similar to small ones; they have relatively stouter bones, and very large mammals stand with their limbs straight, and not flexed and so exposed to bending stresses.

This last point raises a query. If, as is in fact the case, bones are more likely to be broken by bending than by direct compression, is the preceding argument based on direct compression relevant?

Fig. 2a shows the humerus of a mammal in the standing position. Will it break across section XX? This depends on the magnitude of the forces which must be transmitted by the bone at this point. These forces are shown in fig. 2b. By taking moments, $Wh = Td$, or $T = Wh/d$. Now introducing the dimensional argument as before, $W \propto L^3$, $h \propto L$ and $d \propto L$ (the symbol $\propto$ means 'is proportional to'). Hence $T \propto L^3 \times L/L$, or $T \propto L^3$. Now the force T must be transmitted by an area of bone A (see fig. 2c, which shows section XX enlarged).

In other words, a force $T \propto L^3$ must be transitted by an area of bone $A \propto L^2$. Hence bending moments, like direct compression loads, increase with size more rapidly than the capacity of the bones to resist them.

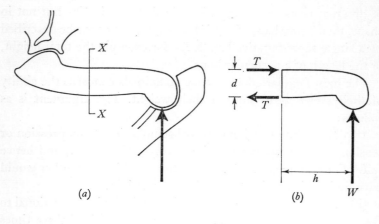

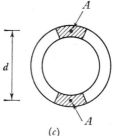

Fig. 2. Bending stresses in the humerus of a mammal.

B. Power output

Less familiar is the way in which power output (work done per unit time: dimensions, force × distance/time) varies with scale. In fact it varies as L^2, and not, as one might at first expect, as L^3: there are three reasons for this.

(i) *Rate of heat loss*

Muscles are devices for turning chemical into mechanical energy. This they do with an efficiency of approximately 25 %; i.e. for every 100 units of chemical energy supplied, 25 appear as mechanical work (force exerted × distance moved) and the remaining 75 as heat. This heat must be lost through the surface, and for a given temperature differential will be dissipated at a rate proportional to L^2. Hence if power output increased as L^3, large animals would overheat.

This is not decisive. Most heat is lost by evaporation of water from the lungs or skin. If heat loss were the only limitation on power output, larger mammals would evolve relatively larger evaporative surfaces.

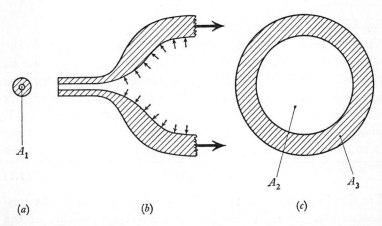

(a)　　　　　　　(b)　　　　　　　(c)

Fig. 3. A diagram of the heart; cut surfaces are shown hatched. (b) is a longitudinal section of part of the ventricle, with the aorta to the left; (a) is a cross-section through the aorta, and (c) is a cross-section through the ventricle.

(ii) *Rate of supply of oxygen*

The rate at which oxygen can be supplied to the tissues depends on the volume of blood reaching them, and this in turn depends on the velocity of blood flow. How will this vary with size?

Fig. 3 shows a diagram of the heart. The maximum force F which can be exerted by the heart muscle per unit cross-sectional area will not vary with size. If the blood pressure in the heart is P (both F and P have dimensions force/area), then $PA_2 = FA_3$, where A_2 and A_3 are the areas shown in the figure. Since F does not vary with size, neither will P. Therefore V, the velocity of flow in the aorta, will not vary with size, because P and V are directly related. (The exact relation between P and V need not worry us; what is important is that a given pressure in the heart will produce a given velocity in the aorta. See example 2.)

The volume of blood delivered by the heart in unit time is proportional to A_1 and hence to L^2. This in turn limits the power output.

Notice that since the volume of the heart is proportional to L^3, the pulse rate will be proportional to $L^2/L^3 = L^{-1}$; this prediction is borne out by observation.

(iii) *Limitations due to stresses in bones and muscles*

When running, muscles do most of their work in overcoming the inertia of the limbs. Thus when the limb is swung fully forwards, it is stationary relative to the body, and has zero kinetic energy. It is then accelerated backwards until the foot has a backwards velocity V relative to the body; the body then has a forwards velocity V relative to the foot and to the ground. To do this, the muscles must do an amount of work equal to the kinetic energy of the leg. Thus from fig. 4,

$$Td = \tfrac{1}{2}mV^2. \tag{1.1}$$

(For simplicity, the mass of the limb has been assumed to be concentrated in the foot; this does not affect the validity of the argument.)

Now T is limited by the tensile strength of muscles and tendons, and hence $T \propto L^2$. Also $d \propto L$, and $m \propto L^3$. Hence substituting in (1.1)

$$L^3 \propto L^3V^2,$$

and hence V does not vary with size.

If t is the time taken for the muscle to contract, then $t \propto L/V \propto L$. Hence the power output of the muscle $= Td/t \propto L^2$.

Much of the kinetic energy of the limb is degraded into heat in the antagonistic muscles during the second half of the stroke. This is the price paid by animals for not having wheels, and explains the advantages of riding a bicycle.

c. Running, jumping, diving, flying

Three reasons have now been given for concluding that the power output of animals is proportional to L^2: the rate at which heat can be dissipated, the rate at which oxygen can be supplied to the tissues,

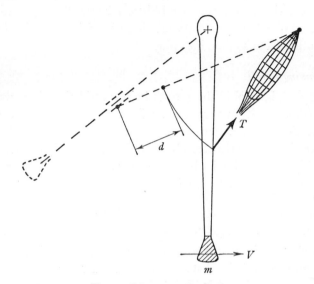

Fig. 4. Diagram of a limb.

and the rate at which work can be done overcoming the inertia of the limbs, all are proportional to L^2. Accepting this conclusion, we can now turn to its implications for other types of performance.

(i) *Running on the flat*

When running on the flat, work is done in overcoming air resistance, and in accelerating the limbs. Some work is also done raising the centre of gravity in animals which progress in a series of leaps; this is considered later.

If a body is moved through the air, the force opposing its motion, or 'drag', is proportional to its surface area and also to the square of the speed, V; i.e. drag $\propto L^2V^2$. Hence the power required to overcome air resistance is proportional to $L^2V^2 \times V = L^2V^3$. The power available is proportional to L^2, and hence we would expect large and small mammals to have the same top speed. The same conclusion emerges if we consider the power required to accelerate the limbs. Thus it was shown above that the power output of the muscles required to overcome the inertia of the limbs when travelling at a given speed is proportional to L^2.

Over the size range from a rabbit to a horse, this conclusion is borne out; speed does not vary consistently with size. Outside that range, other factors come into play.

(ii) *Running uphill*

If when running uphill the rate of increase of height is v, work is done against gravity at a rate proportional to L^3v. If power available is proportional to L^2, then at top speed $L^2 \propto L^3v$, or $v \propto L^{-1}$. In other words, speed up a steep hill should be inversely proportional to size. This conclusion is also borne out; a dog will gallop up a hill which reduces a horse to a walk.

(iii) *Jumping*

Fig. 5 shows three successive stages in a jump. The work done by the muscles is Td; i.e. it is equal to the product of the force exerted on the ground and the distance through which the force moves. Then if the animal has mass m,

$$mgh = Td.$$

T is limited by the mechanical strength of the limb; i.e. $T \propto L^2$, and hence the height jumped,

$$h = \frac{Td}{mg} \propto \frac{L^2 \times L}{L^3}.$$

Hence h does not vary with size. In fact, a jerboa can jump approximately as high as a large kangaroo.

(iv) *Diving*

A diving mammal must carry down with it all the oxygen it needs, either in its lungs, or, as is usually the case in specialised diving mammals, in chemical combination with haemoglobin or myoglobin.

In either case, the volume it can carry is proportional to L^3. The rate of consumption is proportional to L^2. Hence the duration of a dive is proportional to L. This may be one reason why whales are so large.

(v) *Flying*

To determine how the power required to fly varies with size calls for a knowledge of aerodynamics outside the scope of this book. However, the power required for hovering flight can readily be

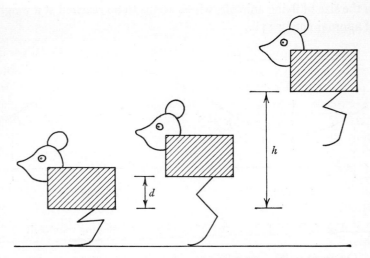

Fig. 5. Diagram of a jumping mammal. The centre picture shows the feet just leaving the ground.

determined. When hovering, a bird produces a downward jet of air, and the momentum of this jet per unit time equals the lift generated, and hence equals the weight of the bird.

Thus let the jet produced have velocity v and cross-sectional area A. The mass of air projected downwards in unit time is then $\rho A v$, where ρ is the air density. If m is the mass of the bird, equating the weight of the bird to the momentum of the jet per unit time gives

$$mg = \rho A v^2. \qquad (1.2)$$

Now $m \propto L^3$ and $A \propto L^2$ (the latter statement is true for birds, but breaks down for small insects, because viscous effects are important to air flow on a small scale). Substituting in (1.2) gives

$$v \propto L^{\frac{1}{2}}.$$

The power output P is used up mainly in generating the jet, and is equal to the kinetic energy in the jet per unit time. Hence

$$P \propto \tfrac{1}{2}\rho A v . v^2 \propto L^{3.5}. \tag{1.3}$$

This conclusion, that the power required to hover is proportional to the 3·5th power of the linear dimensions, holds also for forward flight. Since power available increases as L^2, there is an upper limit to the size of flying animals, which seems to be reached at a weight of approximately 35 lb.

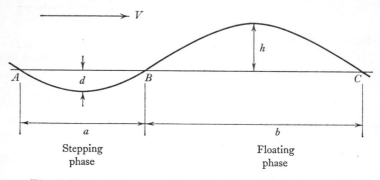

Fig. 6. Path of the centre of gravity of a galloping mammal.

D. Optimal gaits

We now turn to a different problem. When travelling fast, a mammal spends part of the time with all four legs off the ground, and part with one or more legs on the ground. These periods will be called the 'floating' and 'stepping' phases of the gait. The problem to be discussed is how the relative lengths of the floating and stepping phases may be expected to vary with size and speed.

The path of an animal's centre of gravity is shown in fig. 6. During the floating phase (BC) the centre of gravity is accelerating downwards; consequently it must be accelerating upwards during the stepping phase (AB). From fig. 6,

$$d \simeq h \times \frac{a}{b}. \tag{1.4}$$

This equation would be exact if the upward acceleration were uniform during the stepping phase.

The longer the floating phase, the more work the animal must do raising its centre of gravity, but the less often it will have to accelerate its legs. The gait actually adopted will therefore be a compromise. What gait will minimise the power output of an animal of a given size at a given speed? Since this is not the only factor influencing the gait, the answer will correspond only approximately to the gaits actually adopted.

Let the total work done in a single stride be $\overline{W} = W_f + W_s$, where W_f is the work done in raising the centre of gravity and W_s is accelerating the legs. Then

$$W_f = (h+d)\,mg, \tag{1.5}$$

where m is the mass of the animal.

If V is the forward speed, then the time t elapsed between B and the highest point of the floating phase is $b/2V$, and hence

$$h = \tfrac{1}{2}gt^2 = gb^2/8V^2,$$

and substituting for h and d in (1.5), we get

$$W_f = \frac{(a+b)\,bmg^2}{8V^2}. \tag{1.6}$$

The work done accelerating the legs during period AB follows from the fact that while the feet are on the ground they are moving with velocity V relative to the body. If the mass of the whole limb is replaced by an equivalent mass m' at the foot then $W_s = \tfrac{1}{2}m'V^2$. We should at this stage allow for the work done in bringing the foot forwards again. This is quite possible, but it leads to some rather complicated algebra, and for simplicity it will be ignored.

Hence

$$\overline{W} = \frac{(a+b)\,bmg^2}{8V^2} + \tfrac{1}{2}m'V^2. \tag{1.7}$$

The time taken for a complete stride is $(a+b)/V$, and hence the total work done in unit time, $\overline{P}$, is given by

$$\overline{P} = \frac{\overline{W}V}{a+b} = \frac{bmg^2}{8V} + \frac{m'V^3}{2(a+b)}. \tag{1.8}$$

We now write $b = ja$, where j can be regarded as a measure of the 'jumpiness' of the gait. For what value of j is $\bar{P}$ a minimum?

Equation (1.8) becomes

$$\bar{P} = Aj\frac{L^4}{V} + B\frac{V^3L^2}{(1+j)}, \tag{1.9}$$

where V is the forward speed, L a representative linear dimension, and A and B are constants. Differentiating with respect to j, we get

$$\frac{d\bar{P}}{dj} = A\frac{L^4}{V} - B\frac{V^3L^2}{(1+j)^2} = 0 \quad \text{when } \bar{P} \text{ is a minimum.}$$

Hence
$$(1+j)^2 = \frac{B}{A}\frac{V^4}{L^2},$$

or
$$1 + j \propto V^2/L. \tag{1.10}$$

From (1.10) we conclude that j increases with V (compare walk, trot, gallop) and decreases with L. In fact at top speed, j is zero for an elephant, 0·3 for a horse and 1 for a greyhound, approximately. But j does not alter as rapidly with L as (1.10) would suggest, presumably because minimisation of power output is not the only criterion determining gaits.

Examples

1 The rate at which a substance diffuses across a surface is proportional to the area of the surface and to the concentration gradient normal to the surface. For animals without a circulation system, how would you expect muscular power output to vary with size?

2 It was stated that the velocity of blood in the aorta is directly related to the difference in pressure between the heart and arteries. Satisfy yourself of this, and find the relationship, by equating the work done by the heart muscle to the kinetic energy of the arterial blood.

3 Desert animals may have to travel long distances between water-holes. How do you think the maximum distance travelled would vary with the size of the animal?

4 A planet has two-thirds earth's gravity, and an atmospheric density half that of the earth, but with the same oxygen tension.

How heavy would the heaviest flying animals be, if 35 lb. is the maximum on earth? Supposing a greyhound could adjust its gait on this planet to minimise its power output, for what proportion of the time would all four legs be off the ground when travelling at a speed equal to its top speed on earth?

5   Speculate on the reasons limiting the maximum size of animals swimming by means of cilia. (*Hint*: why do you suppose cilia in invertebrate larvae are often confined to narrow tracts?)

2 POPULATION REGULATION: GENERATIONS SEPARATE

A. Introduction

It is often the case that the number of animals of a given species in a given area either remains approximately constant from year to year, or fluctuates with a rather regular periodicity about some intermediate value. In this and the next chapter, some of the factors which may regulate animal numbers, and which may be responsible for fluctuations, are discussed.

Any attempt to formulate the problem mathematically necessarily leaves out many relevant factors. The attempt is nevertheless illuminating, for two reasons. First, it provides a rapid way of discovering the kind of effect various features—for example predation, parasitism, territorial behaviour, a long or short period of immaturity—may have on the behaviour of a population. Second, it suggests what needs to be measured before the behaviour of any particular species can be understood.

B. Reproduction rate constant

Suppose there is a species of animal which has a single breeding season during the summer, and in which adults which breed in one summer die before the next.

Let $X_1, X_2, X_3 \ldots X_n \ldots$ be the numbers of adult females at the start of the breeding season in the first, second, third ... nth ... year.

Let each female produce, on the average, R female offspring which survive to breed in the next year.

Then
$$X_{n+1} = RX_n. \tag{2.1}$$

This is a 'recurrence relation', which tells us what the population will be next year in terms of the population this year.

It can be written in a different way, by expressing the *change* in the population in one year, i.e.

$$\Delta X_n = X_{n+1} - X_n,$$

and then obviously $\quad \Delta X_n = (R-1)X_n.$ $\qquad$ (2.2)

In general, R will depend on X; for example when the population is large, there may not be enough food to go round, and so R may be small. But we will first consider the case when R is a constant. Thus we want to solve the equation

$$X_{n+1} = RX_n.$$

By 'solving' this equation, we mean finding X as a function of the generation n, and of the 'initial conditions'—in this case X_1, the size of the population in the first generation. Finding solutions of recurrence relations usually consists of guessing an answer and then showing that the answer fits; in this respect it is like integration.

In this case, it is fairly easy to guess that the answer will be of the form

$$X_n = a\lambda^n,$$

where a and λ are unknown constants.

Then substituting in the equation, we have

$$a\lambda^{n+1} = Ra\lambda^n \quad \text{or} \quad \lambda = R.$$

Whence $\qquad X_n = aR^n.$

We find a from the initial conditions. Thus

$$X_1 = aR \quad \text{or} \quad a = \frac{X_1}{R},$$

and hence the solution is

$$X_n = \frac{X_1}{R}.R^n \quad \text{or} \quad X_n = X_1 R^{n-1}. \qquad (2.3)$$

Whence, knowing the initial size of the population, the reproductive rate R and the number of generations, we can find the population size. Thus for example if $n = 4$, $X_1 = 1$ and $R = 2$,

$$X = 1 \times 2^3 = 8.$$

Had we wished we could have calculated this arithmetically from (2.2) by iteration, thus:

n	1		2		3		4
X	1		2		4		8
ΔX		1		2		4	

There is no point in doing this iteration when the equation can be solved algebraically, as it can in this case, but the method will be useful later on.

Returning to (2.3), it is clear that if $R > 1$ the population will increase without limit, and if $R < 1$ it will decrease to zero.

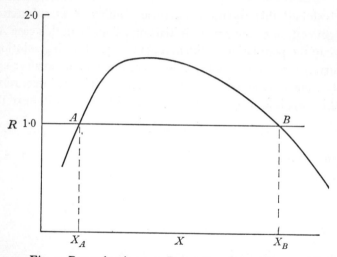

Fig. 7. Reproductive rate R as a function of density X.

c. Density-dependent reproduction

In general, R will depend on X. A possible type of dependance is shown in fig. 7.

If the population is to survive at all, there must be some range of values for which $R > 1$. In general, when X is very large, R will become less than one. In some species, if X is too small R may again become less than one, perhaps because females do not find mates; such an effect has been shown in the figure.

When $R = 1$ (i.e. at points A and B) the population will just reproduce itself with constant numbers X_A or X_B; these are points of *equilibrium*. It is fairly easy to see that B is a point of *stable* equilibrium; thus if X rises above X_B, $R < 1$ and the population will decrease, and if X falls below X_B, $R > 1$ and the population will increase. By a similar argument, A is a point of unstable equilibrium. If X falls below X_A the population will become extinct.

We would like to know more about the behaviour of the population in the region of the stable equilibrium point X_B: for example, does it oscillate either side of X_B, and if so do the oscillations decrease in amplitude with time? It is not very difficult to see the answer to these questions, but we will answer them by using a trick which is often helpful for investigating small displacements near an equilibrium point—whether in chemistry, population dynamics or economics.

The trick is illustrated in fig. 8.

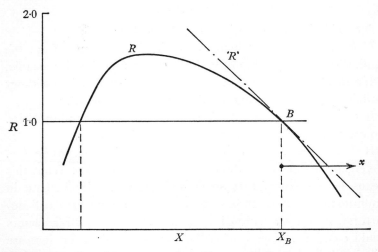

Fig. 8. The linearising assumption. For small displacements from the equilibrium value X_B, the true value of R can be replaced by the straight line, 'R'.

First, we write $X = X_B + x$; i.e. we measure population size not absolutely (X), but as a departure, x, from the equilibrium. Note that whereas X is necessarily positive, x can be positive or negative.

Second, we replace the actual graph of R vs. X with a straight line which has the same slope at the equilibrium point X_B.

Since when $x = 0$, $R = 1$, the equation of this line is

$$R = 1 - bx,$$

where $-b$ is the slope of the line.

Equation (2.1) now becomes

$$X_{n+1} = (1 - bx_n) X_n.$$
$$\therefore \quad X_B + x_{n+1} = (1 - bx_n)(X_B + x_n)$$
$$= X_B + x_n - bX_B x_n - bx_n^2.$$

Now for *small* displacements, x_n^2 can be ignored in comparison with x_n, and hence

$$x_{n+1} = x_n - bX_B x_n,$$

and writing $bX_B = K$, a constant, we have

$$x_{n+1} = (1 - K)x_n, \tag{2.4}$$

or

$$\Delta x_n = -Kx_n.$$

A consideration of equation (2.4) shows that:

If K negative (i.e. R increases with X), departures from the equilibrium increase without limit; i.e. the equilibrium is unstable.

If $0 < K < 1$, the population approaches the equilibrium without oscillations; in engineering terminology, it is 'damped'.

If $1 < K < 2$, there are oscillations of decreasing amplitude (i.e. 'convergent' oscillations) about the equilibrium point.

If $K > 2$, there are oscillations of increasing amplitude (i.e. 'divergent' oscillations) about the equilibrium point. What this means in practice is that small oscillations would increase in amplitude. The assumptions made hold true only for small departures. As the oscillation increased in amplitude, other factors would come into play, so that the amplitude might not increase indefinitely.

These statements about the behaviour of equation (2.4) for different values of K can easily be seen to be true by substituting various values of K and calculating what happens. For example, if $K = 1 \cdot 5$,

n	1	2	3	4	
x	1	$-0 \cdot 5$	$0 \cdot 25$	$-0 \cdot 125$	
Δx	$-1 \cdot 5$	$+0 \cdot 75$	$-0 \cdot 375$		and so on.

Alternatively, by comparison with (2.1) and (2.3), we can see that the solution of equation (2.4) is

$$x_n = x_1(1 - K)^{n-1},$$

and the same conclusions follow.

The conclusion that emerges is that too 'strong' a regulation (i.e. K large) may lead to oscillations.

D. Delayed regulation

It is possible that the reproductive rate R may depend, not only on the population density at the time, but on the population density in the past. For example, the reproduction of a herbivorous species will depend on the vegetation, which may in turn depend on how much of the vegetation was eaten by herbivores in the previous year.

To gain some idea of the effect of such a delay in the effects of population density on its own increase, a much over-simplified example will be considered. It will be assumed that R depends only on the population density in the previous year, and not on the immediate density nor on the density in still earlier years. In mathematics, the shorthand way of writing 'R depends only on the population density in the previous year' is '$R = f(X_{n-1})$', or 'R is a function of X_{n-1}'. By saying this, we mean that if we knew enough we could draw a graph of R against X_{n-1}, just as in fig. 7 we drew a graph of R against X.

Thus $$X_{n+1} = RX_n,$$
where $$R = f(X_{n-1}),$$
which can be rewritten

$$X_{n+2} = X_{n+1}f(X_n) \qquad (2.5)$$

If we know the form of $f(X)$, this equation can easily be solved by iteration. In general, an analytical solution cannot be found. But as in the case considered in the last section, we can investigate small displacements from the equilibrium density X_E.

Thus if we write $X_n = X_E + x_n$, then when $x_n = 0$, $f(X_n) = 1$. If we assume that for small displacements the graph of R against X_n is a straight line, then so is the graph of R against x_n, and hence $f(X_n) \simeq 1 - bx_n$, and so for small displacements:

$$X_E + x_{n+2} = (X_E + x_{n+1})(1 - bx_n),$$

or ignoring the term in $x_n.x_{n+1}$, and writing $bX_E = k$,

$$x_{n+2} - x_{n+1} + kx_n = 0. \qquad (2.6)$$

This equation should be compared with (2.4) which can be written

$$x_{n+1} = x_n - Kx_n,$$

whereas (2.6) is equivalent to

$$x_{n+1} = x_n - kx_{n-1}.$$

They differ in that in (2.6) there is a delay of one generation in the 'regulative' term kx_{n-1}.

Before finding an algebraic solution of (2.6) some idea of its behaviour can be obtained by arithmetical iteration, assuming $k = 1 \cdot 5$; remember that when $K = 1 \cdot 5$, (2.4) gave a convergent oscillation. Before iterating, we have to take as initial conditions two successive values of x; we will assume $x_1 = x_2 = 1$. Then:

generation	1	2	3	4	5	6	7	8	9
x	1	1	$-0 \cdot 5$	$-2 \cdot 0$	$-1 \cdot 25$	$+1 \cdot 75$	$+3 \cdot 62$	$+0 \cdot 99$	$-4 \cdot 43$
$\Delta x = -kx_{n-1}$			$-1 \cdot 5$	$-1 \cdot 5$	$+0 \cdot 75$	$+3$	$+1 \cdot 87$	$-2 \cdot 63$	$-5 \cdot 42$

and it is apparent that this is a divergent oscillation. The transformation of a convergent into a divergent oscillation by a delay in the feed-back loop is of common occurrence.

It would be possible to find the values of k for which convergent and divergent oscillations occur by a process of arithmetical trial and error. But it is quicker to find an analytical solution of (2.6). The solution of such equations is discussed in appendix 4. By analogy with (2.2), we guess the solution $x_n = A\lambda^n$. Then

$$A\lambda^{n+2} - A\lambda^{n+1} + kA\lambda^n = 0.$$

$$\therefore \quad \lambda^2 - \lambda + k = 0,$$

an equation which has two solutions:

$$\lambda_1 = \frac{1}{2} + \frac{\sqrt{(1-4k)}}{2}; \quad \lambda_2 = \frac{1}{2} - \frac{\sqrt{(1-4k)}}{2}.$$

Hence the complete solution of (2.6) is

$$x_n = A\left[\frac{1}{2} + \frac{\sqrt{(1-4k)}}{2}\right]^n + B\left[\frac{1}{2} - \frac{\sqrt{(1-4k)}}{2}\right]^n, \qquad (2.7)$$

where A and B are constants which can be chosen to fit the initial conditions.

Clearly if either value of λ is greater than 1, the equilibrium is unstable. But this can only be the case if k is negative—i.e. if fertility increases as the population grows.

If $0 < k < \frac{1}{4}$, both values of λ lie between 0 and 1, and the equilibrium is stable and non-oscillatory.

If $k > \frac{1}{4}$, then $\sqrt{(1-4k)}$ is imaginary. It is shown in Appendix 4 that in this case (2.7) can be re-written,

$$x_n = k^{\frac{1}{2}n}[\alpha \cos n\theta + \beta \sin n\theta], \qquad (2.8)$$

where $\theta = \cos^{-1}\left(\dfrac{1}{2\sqrt{k}}\right)$, and α and β are constants. This is an oscillation which increases in amplitude with increasing n if $k > 1$.

We can now compare the behaviour of (2.4) and (2.6), as follows:

	No delay	1 generation delay
equilibrium unstable	K negative	k negative
stable equilibrium, no oscillation	$0 < K < 1$	$0 < k < \frac{1}{4}$
convergent oscillation	$1 < K < 2$	$\frac{1}{4} < k < 1$
divergent oscillation	$K > 2$	$k > 1$

E. The logistic equation

Returning to equation (2.1), we will now seek for a more plausible relationship between R and X. We will assume that there is some equilibrium number, X_E, and we will also assume that the further the actual population number falls short of this equilibrium number, the more rapidly it grows. More precisely, we will assume that

$$\frac{X_{n+1} - X_n}{X_n} \propto (X_E - X_n). \qquad (2.9)$$

The left-hand side of this relation measures the population growth in one year, as a fraction of the population size in that year; it is in effect a rate of interest. The right-hand side measures the difference between the actual population size and its equilibrium value. The assumption that these two measures are proportional to one another leads to the 'logistic' equation, although the term is usually confined to the continuous case considered in the next chapter.

Relation (2.9) can be written

$$X_{n+1} - X_n = c(X_E - X_n)X_n$$

or
$$X_{n+1} = (cX_E + 1 - cX_n)X_n. \tag{2.10}$$

Thus the maximum reproductive rate, when X_n is small, is $R_{max} = cX_E + 1$.

To get some idea of how this equation behaves, consider a simple case when the maximum rate of increase is fairly small, i.e. when $R_{max} = 4$.

Then $cX_E = 3$, and taking, for example, an equilibrium density $X_E = 60$, then $c = 1/20$. Suppose the initial population size $X_1 = 50$, then iterating:

generation	1	2	3	4	5	6	7	8
X_n	50	75	18·7	57·4	64·9	49·0	76·0	15·2
$X_E - X_n$	10	−15	41·3	2·6	−4·9	11	−16	
ΔX†		25	−56·3	+38·7	+7·5	−15·9	+27·0	−60·8

$$\dagger \ \Delta X = \tfrac{1}{20}(X_E - X_n)X_n$$

In this case, the population fluctuates irregularly about its equilibrium value of 60. This could have been foreseen. Thus although it is not easy to guess a solution to equation (2.10), it is easy to investigate the behaviour close to the equilibrium point. As before, let $X_n = X_E + x_n$. Then

$$\Delta x = c(X_E - X_n)X_n = -cX_n . x_n$$
$$= -cX_E x_n - cx_n^2,$$

or for small displacements,

$$\Delta x = -cX_E x_n.$$

And, as in §C, if $cX_E > 2$, this gives a divergent oscillation. The amplitude does not in practice increase indefinitely, because when x_n is large, x_n^2 cannot be ignored.

If $R_{max} < 2$, and hence $cX_E < 1$, the population will approach its equilibrium density without oscillations.

If R_{max} lies between 2 and 3, oscillations will be convergent.

F. Predator–Prey

It is now possible to analyse the relations between a predator and prey species.

Let X_n and Y_n be the numbers of prey and predator respectively.

Suppose first that in the absence of the predator, the prey species is limited by some other factor to a density of X_E, and that its population obeys the logistic relation

$$\Delta X_n = cX_E X_n - cX_n^2.$$

In the presence of the predator, this equation should be modified by a term allowing for the individuals killed by predators. This term could take a number of forms. For example, if there were an amount of 'cover' capable of protecting a limited number of prey, and if those prey unable to occupy this cover were killed, then all prey above some fixed number would be killed. Or suppose that the predator is rare, and limited by some factor other than the abundance of this particular prey (e.g. by the abundance of some other prey species). Each predator might then take a fixed quantity of prey regardless of the abundance of the prey. In this case this relevant term would be $-CY_n$, where C is a constant.

A more interesting case is the one in which the abundance of the predator is limited by the abundance of the prey. This requires that the number of prey taken by each predator must decrease as the abundance of the prey decreases; if this were not the case, changes in prey abundance could have no regulating influence on the predator. (A conceivable alternative is that each predator takes a fixed quantity of prey, but that as the prey becomes less abundant, the predators must spend an increasing proportion of their time searching, and so have less time for successful reproduction.)

A simple assumption is that each predator kills a number of prey proportional to the abundance of the prey, and hence

$$\Delta x_n = cX_E X_n - cX_n^2 - CX_n Y_n. \tag{2.11}$$

This assumption would be true if each predator searched a constant area, the areas searched by different predators not overlapping, and found a constant proportion of the prey in that area.

We now want an equation for Y_n. One plausible assumption is that the number of offspring produced by each predator is proportional to the number of prey killed by that predator; this is to assume a constant 'conversion efficiency' in turning ingested food into offspring. Now the number of prey killed by each predator is CX_n, and so the number of offspring produced by each predator is equal to

$$\text{Constant}.CX_n = KX_n \quad \text{say.}$$

Hence
$$Y_{n+1} = KX_n Y_n. \tag{2.12}$$

It is easier to interpret the solution of equations (2.11) and (2.12) if we express them in terms of R and r, the maximum reproductive rates of the prey and predator respectively.

Thus R is the rate of increase of the prey when it is rare, and in the absence of the predator. From page 26, $R = cX_E + 1$, and hence $c = (R-1)/X_E$.

Substituting in (2.11) gives

$$\Delta X_n = (R-1) X_n - (R-1) X_n^2/X_E - CX_n Y_n$$

or
$$X_{n+1} = RX_n - (R-1) X_n^2/X_E - CX_n Y_n. \tag{2.13}$$

Suppose now that the prey are at their equilibrium density X_E in the absence of predators, and that a few predators are then introduced; let the initial rate of increase of the predators be r. Then from (2.12)

$$r = Y_{n+1}/Y_n = KX_E,$$

and so (2.12) becomes

$$Y_{n+1} = rX_n Y_n/X_E. \tag{2.14}$$

The first stage in investigating equations (2.13) and (2.14) will be to study a particular numerical example.

Let $R = 1\cdot5$; with this value, the prey species by itself, in the absence of predators, would approach its equilibrium density X_E without oscillation.

Let $X_E = 100$. This choice has no significance—it amounts merely to a choice of the unit area.

We will suppose that when $X_n = X_E$, each predator kills 50 prey; hence $CX_E = 50$, or $C = 0\cdot5$. We will also suppose that this diet is sufficient to enable the predator to double in numbers each year; i.e. $r = 2$.

The equations then become:

$$\left.\begin{array}{l} X_{n+1} = (1\cdot5 - X_n/200 - Y_n/2) X_n, \\ Y_{n+1} = \frac{1}{50}X_n Y_n. \end{array}\right\}$$

At equilibrium, when both predators and prey just maintain themselves:

$$\tfrac{1}{50}Xn = 1 \quad \text{or} \quad X_n = 50,$$
$$1\cdot5 - \frac{Xn}{200} - \frac{Yn}{2} = 1 \quad \text{or} \quad Yn = 0\cdot5.$$

The equations can easily be iterated. Starting with the prey at their equilibrium density, $X_1 = 50$, and the predator relatively rare, $Y_1 = 0\cdot2$, the results of iteration are shown in fig. 9. The result is an oscillation of long period, whose amplitude varies little with time.

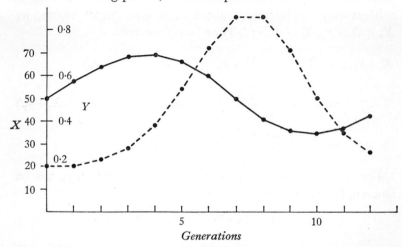

Fig. 9. The numbers of prey, X, (full line) and of predators, Y, (broken line) in successive generations, for the imaginary example described in the text.

Equations (2.13) and (2.14) can be investigated algebraically. The procedure is a little complicated, and it will help to follow the details if the various stages are summarised first. They are as follows:

(i) The equilibrium values of X and Y are found.

(ii) New equations are derived for small displacements about these equilibrium values.

(iii) One of the variables is eliminated from these equations; in much the same way, the first step in solving simple simultaneous equations is to eliminate one of the variables.

(iv) The resulting equation has the form considered in appendix 4.

If X_s, Y_s are the equilibrium values of X and Y (we cannot use X_E and Y_E because we have already used X_E for the equilibrium value of X in the absence of predators), then

from (2.14) $\qquad Y_s = rX_sY_s/X_E \quad \text{or} \quad X_s = X_E/r,$

from (2.13) $\qquad 1 = R - \dfrac{(R-1)X_s}{rX_s} - CY_s$

or $\qquad Y_s = \dfrac{1}{C}\left(R - 1 - \dfrac{R-1}{r}\right).$

Measuring displacements about these equilibrium values, let $X_n = X_s + x_n$, $Y_n = Y_s + y_n$. Then (2.13) becomes

$$X_s + x_{n+1} = \left\{R - \frac{R-1}{rX_s}(X_s + x_n) - C(Y_s + y_n)\right\}(X_s + x_n)$$

$$= \left\{R - \frac{R-1}{r} - \frac{(R-1)x_n}{rX_s} - R + \frac{R-1}{r} + 1 - Cy_n\right\}(X_s + x_n)$$

$$= \left\{1 - \frac{(R-1)x_n}{rX_s} - Cy_n\right\}(X_s + x_n).$$

For small displacements, when terms in x_n^2 and $x_n y_n$ can be ignored, this reduces to

$$X_s + x_{n+1} = X_s + x_n - \frac{(R-1)x_n}{r} - CX_s y_n$$

or $\qquad x_{n+1} = x_n\left(1 - \dfrac{R-1}{r}\right) - \dfrac{CX_E}{r}y_n, \qquad (2.15)$

and equation (2.14) becomes

$$Y_s + y_{n+1} = \frac{r}{X_E}(X_s + x_n)(Y_s + y_n)$$

$$= \frac{r}{X_E}\left\{\frac{X_E\,Y_s}{r} + \frac{X_E y_n}{r} + x_n\,Y_s + x_n y_n\right\},$$

and ignoring the term in $x_n y_n$, this becomes

$$Y_s + y_{n+1} = Y_s + y_n + \frac{r\,Y_s x_n}{X_E}$$

$$\therefore \quad y_{n+1} = y_n + \frac{r}{CX_E}\left(R - 1 - \frac{R-1}{r}\right)x_n. \qquad (2.16)$$

We now have to eliminate one of the variables, x_n and y_n. From (2.16),

$$x_n = \frac{y_{n+1} - y_n}{\alpha}$$

and hence

$$x_{n+1} = \frac{y_{n+2} - y_{n+1}}{\alpha},$$

where

$$\alpha = \frac{r}{CX_E}\left(R - 1 - \frac{R-1}{r}\right).$$

Substituting in (2.15), this gives

$$\frac{y_{n+2} - y_{n+1}}{\alpha} = \frac{y_{n+1} - y_n}{\alpha}\left(1 - \frac{R-1}{r}\right) - \frac{CX_E}{r}y_n,$$

and after rearrangement, this reduces to

$$y_{n+2} - y_{n+1}\left[2 - \frac{R-1}{r}\right] + y_n\left[R - \frac{2(R-1)}{r}\right] = 0. \qquad (2.17)$$

This is a recurrence relation of the form considered in appendix 4. It gives y_n in terms of the maximum reproductive rates R and r of the prey and predator respectively. It is easier to handle if we write $(R-1)/2r = \beta$. Then

$$y_{n+2} - 2(1 - \beta)y_{n+1} + (R - 4\beta)y_n = 0. \qquad (2.18)$$

The solution of this equation is

$$y_n = A\lambda_1^n + B\lambda_2^n, \qquad (2.19)$$

where

$$\lambda_1 = 1 - \beta + \sqrt{[(1 + \beta)^2 - R]}; \quad \lambda_2 = 1 - \beta - \sqrt{[(1 + \beta)^2 - R]};$$

and A and B are constants.

Unfortunately, having found a solution, it is not immediately obvious what it means. Clearly, the behaviour of y_n depends on the values of λ_1 and λ_2. We proceed as follows:

(i) $R > (1 + \beta)^2$. λ_1 and λ_2 are complex. (2.20)

It is shown in appendix 4 that in this case (2.19) describes an oscillation, which is divergent if $R - 4\beta > 1$: i.e. if

$$R > 1 + 4\beta. \qquad (2.21)$$

(ii) $R < (1+\beta)^2$. λ_1 and λ_2 are real.

(a) If $\lambda_1 > 1$, y_n increases without limit as n increases. This will happen if

$$1 - \beta + \sqrt{[(1+\beta)^2 - R]} > 1,$$

which reduces to $1 + 2\beta > R$, or substituting for β, to $r < 1$.

But if $r < 1$, the predator will rapidly become extinct, and no equilibrium can exist.

(b) If $\lambda_2 < 0$, the system will oscillate: i.e. if

$$1 - \beta - \sqrt{[(1+\beta)^2 - R]} < 0,$$

$$\text{or} \quad \sqrt{[(1+\beta)^2 - R]} > 1 - \beta.$$

Since $R < (1+\beta)^2$, this must be true if $\beta > 1$.
If $\beta < 1$, then

$$(1+\beta)^2 - R > (1-\beta)^2 \quad \text{or} \quad R < 4\beta.$$

Thus the system oscillates if

$$\beta > 1 \quad \text{or if} \quad R < 4\beta. \tag{2.22}$$

(c) If $\lambda_2 < -1$, the oscillations will be divergent: i.e. if

$$1 - \beta - \sqrt{[(1+\beta)^2 - R]} < -1,$$

and proceeding as before, the oscillations are divergent if

$$\beta > 2 \quad \text{or} \quad R < 6\beta - 3. \tag{2.23}$$

Inequalities (2.20–23) are summarised in fig. 10. Remembering that $\beta = (R-1)/2r$, this can be converted into fig. 11, which enables us to predict the behaviour of the predator–prey system from a knowledge of R and r, the maximum reproductive rates of prey and predator respectively. Notice that in our numerical example, $R = 1.5$ and $r = 2$, and we would expect an oscillation of constant amplitude, which is what we found.

Except when R and r are both small, the system oscillates with increasing amplitude.

In region B (R large, r small) the prey would oscillate in the absence of the predator. The predator oscillates because the prey are oscillating, but is not the cause of the oscillations. This corresponds to the Canadian game cycle; the foxes and lynxes oscillate

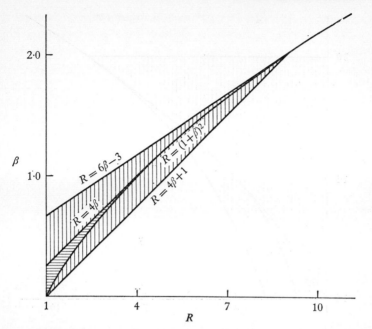

Fig. 10. The behaviour of a predator and prey. A particular pair of species can be represented by a point on the diagram; R is the reproductive rate of the prey in the absence of predators, and $\beta = (R-1)/2r$, where r is the reproductive rate of the predator as defined in the text. In the horizontally hatched area, the system does not oscillate; in the vertically hatched area, there is a convergent oscillation; in the unhatched area, there is a divergent oscillation.

because the rabbits do. In fact, the presence of predators may prevent oscillations; in region C, oscillations are damped, although in the absence of predators they would be divergent.

In region A (R small, r large) the predator can be regarded as responsible for the oscillations, since in their absence the oscillations would cease. Whether such divergent oscillations would lead to the extinction first of prey and then of the predator depends on what other factors come into play. For example, the prey might be saved from extinction if a limited amount of 'cover' existed, so that the prey had a better chance of survival when rare; the predator might be saved from extinction if an alternative prey species existed.

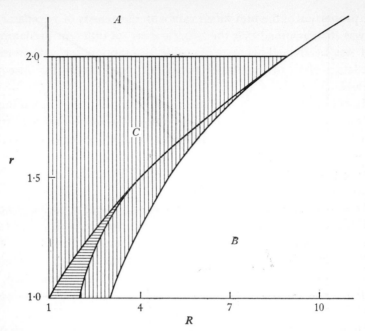

Fig. 11. The behaviour of a predator and prey. This figure presents the same information as fig. 10, but directly in terms of the reproductive rates R and r.

G. Host–Parasitoid

A case of interaction between species for which it is possible to write down the equations with a fair degree of plausibility has been considered theoretically by Nicholson and Bailey, and has been tested observationally by Varley. It concerns the case of a host insect attacked by a specific 'parasitoid'—i.e. an insect such as an ichneumon or chalcid which is free-living as an adult and which lays eggs in the larvae of the host. The particular case considered is that in which either only a single egg is laid per host larva or, if more than one egg is laid, only one survives. This leads to the mathematically simple situation that a single host larva can give rise either to one host adult, or to one parasitoid adult.

The first problem to be solved is how the proportion of host larvae to be parasitised will vary with the density of the parasite. This is similar to the question asked in the last section, i.e. how does the proportion of the prey killed vary with the density of a predator. It was then assumed that the 'search areas' of different predators did not overlap. This is a plausible assumption for vertebrate predators showing territorial behaviour, but hardly for insect parasitoids.

It will be assumed that each parasitoid searches an area a, finding all the hosts in that area. The assumption is exactly equivalent in this case to the assumption that each searches an area ka $(k > 1)$ and finds a proportion $1/k$ of the hosts. Thus a is the 'effective' search area. It can be any shape, and can overlap with the areas searched by other individuals.

In some area A, large relative to a, let the number of parasites be AY (i.e. Y is the population density of the parasite). We want to know the probability that some particular host individual in area A will be parasitised. As is often the case, it is easier to calculate in the first instance the probability that the individual is not parasitised.

The probability that the host individual is parasitised by one particular parasite in the area is clearly a/A.

Hence the probability that the host is *not* parasitised by that particular parasite is $1 - a/A$.

Now there are AY parasites in the area, and if each of them searches independently (i.e. there is no dividing up of the search area between them), the probability that the host individual is not parasitised by any parasite is

$$(1 - a/A)^{AY}.$$

In this expression, a/A is small and AY is large. We are therefore interested in a simpler expression for $(1 - x)^N$, where x is small and N large. It is shown in appendix 6 that in such a case $(1 - x)^N \simeq e^{-Nx}$, and hence $(1 - a/A)^{AY} \simeq e^{-aY}$.

Thus a fraction e^{-aY} of the host individuals are un-parasitised, and a fraction $1 - e^{-aY}$ are parasitised at least once.

If at the start of the breeding season the density of female parasites is Y and of female hosts is X, and if on the average each female host lays $2R$ eggs which survive to pupate, then after parasitisation, the density of pupae containing hosts is $2RXe^{-aY}$, and containing parasites is $2RX(1 - e^{-aY})$.

Assuming a fraction S of these hosts and parasites survive to breed in the next season (it is reasonable to assume the same value of S for host and parasite if both over-winter in the host pupae), and assuming a $1:1$ sex ratio for both species, we have

$$Y_{n+1} = RSX_n(1 - e^{-aY_n}) \quad \text{and} \quad X_{n+1} = RSX_n e^{-aY_n},$$

or writing $RS = k$

$$Y_{n+1} = kX_n(1 - e^{-aY_n}) \tag{2.24}$$

and

$$X_{n+1} = kX_n e^{-aY_n}. \tag{2.25}$$

The procedure for solving these equations is identical to that adopted for equations (2.12) and (2.13).

We first find the equilibrium values X_E and Y_E: from (2.25)

$$ke^{-aY_E} = 1 \quad \text{or} \quad Y_E = \frac{1}{a}\ln k,$$

and substituting in (2.24):

$$\frac{1}{a}\ln k = kX_E\left(1 - \frac{1}{k}\right) \quad \text{or} \quad X_E = \frac{\ln k}{a(k-1)}.$$

Next we consider small departures from the equilibrium. Let $X_n = X_E + x_n$, $Y_n = Y_E + y_n$. Equation (2.25) then becomes

$$X_E + x_{n+1} = k(X_E + x_n)e^{-a(Y_E + y_n)}$$

$$= kX_E e^{-aY_E}e^{-ay_n} + kx_n e^{-aY_E}e^{-ay_n},$$

and when y_n is small, $e^{-ay_n} \simeq 1 - ay_n$, and remembering that $ke^{-aY_E} = 1$, this becomes

$$X_E + x_{n+1} = X_E(1 - ay_n) + x_n(1 - ay_n),$$

and hence, ignoring the term in $x_n y_n$,

$$x_{n+1} = -aX_E y_n + x_n$$

or

$$x_{n+1} = x_n - \frac{\ln k}{k-1}y_n \tag{2.26}$$

and by a similar calculation

$$y_{n+1} = y_n + (k-1)x_n. \tag{2.27}$$

We now eliminate one of the variables. Thus from (2.26),

$$y_n = \frac{k-1}{\ln k}(x_n - x_{n+1}),$$

and substituting this in (2.27) gives

$$\frac{(k-1)}{\ln k}(x_{n+1} - x_{n+2}) = \frac{(k-1)}{\ln k}(x_n - x_{n+1}) + (k-1)x_n,$$

or
$$x_{n+2} - 2x_{n+1} + (1 + \ln k)x_n = 0. \qquad (2.28)$$

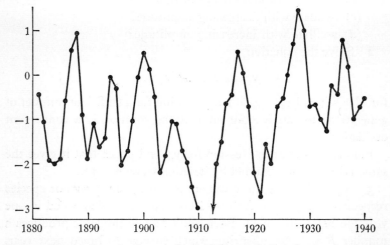

Fig. 12. Fluctuations in the numbers of the moth *Bupalus* in pine forests in Germany, on a logarithmic scale. The ordinate is $\log_{10} x$, where x is the number of pupae per sq.m. Thus there are fluctuations of the order of a thousand-fold in density, with a periodicity of about 6 years prior to 1906, and a somewhat longer period subsequently. Parasitism may be part of the explanation for these oscillations. (After Varley, G. C. (1949). *J. An. Ecol.* **18**, 117.)

This equation is solved in exactly the same way as equations (2.6) and (2.17). It gives an oscillation, which is divergent if $1 + \ln k > 1$.

Now k is necessarily greater than 1; it is the annual rate of increase of the host in the absence of the parasitoid. Hence $\ln k$ is positive, and $1 + \ln k > 1$.

The conclusion is that host–parasitoid relations, when it is assumed that the host density is limited only by the parasitoid, and that the parasitoid is confined to one host species, lead to oscillations of large amplitude. This conclusion has been used by Varley to explain fluctuations in the numbers of various species of moths in pine forests (see fig. 12).

Examples

1 If $x_{n+2} + Cx_{n+1} + Cx_n = 0$, and n is large and increasing, for what range of values of C does x_n

    (a) increase without change of sign?

    (b) decrease without change of sign?

    (c) oscillate with decreasing amplitude?

    (d) oscillate with increasing amplitude?

2 Solve the equation

$$y_{n+2} - y_{n+1} + Ky_n = 0$$

for $K = 0.5$ and $y_1 = y_2 = 1$ by iteration for a sufficient number of generations to satisfy yourself that the solution is a convergent oscillation.

Find an algebraic expression for y_n, and check that it gives the same value as you obtained by iteration when $n = 10$.

3 X_n and Y_n are the numbers of a prey and predator species respectively in year n. Adults of both species which breed in one year die before the next. Each adult female predator produces a number $R = X_n/20$ offspring which survive to breed next year. Each adult female prey produces $R' = 6/Y_n$ offspring which survive to breed next year.

    (a) Find the equilibrium numbers of prey and predator.

    (b) Write down an equation similar to (2.17) for small departures from this equilibrium.

    (c) What is the behaviour of this equation?

    (d) How does the behaviour depend on the choice of 20 and 6 in the equations for R and R'?

    (e) What generalisation are you tempted to draw from this example?

3 POPULATION REGULATION: GENERATIONS NOT SEPARATE

So far we have considered species with an annual breeding season, and have assumed that individuals breeding in one summer die before the next, so that generations are 'separate', members of one generation never breeding with members of another. The appropriate mathematical formulation for such cases was in the form of a recurrence relation. We will now turn to the case where the population breeds continuously; the appropriate mathematical descriptions will then be differential equations.

Let the population density at time t be x. To start with, we will make the artificial assumption that the rate of change of the population density, dx/dt, depends only on conditions at time t, and does not depend on the past history of the population. This assumption is artificial, among other reasons, because it ignores the age structure of the population. Thus if, for example, the food supply to a population were suddenly increased, there might be a rapid increase in the rate at which adult females in the population laid eggs, but there would be an inevitable delay before these eggs hatched into feeding individuals, and a larger delay before they developed into adults themselves capable of breeding. Thus an adequate description of the population requires a knowledge, not only of the total numbers, but of the numbers in each age group. And since the number in, for example, the 30-day-old group depends on conditions 30 days ago, an adequate description cannot ignore past history.

The consequences of population age structure are considered below, but for the time being they are ignored. The resulting description will apply most nearly to micro-organisms reproducing by binary fission, although even for them it is not wholly adequate.

A. Logarithmic growth

Consider first a species with an unlimited food supply, and without predators or competitors.

In any time interval δt, an individual chosen at random has a probability $a\,\delta t$ of giving rise to a new individual. In a population reproducing by binary fission with a time between successive fissions of T, $a = 1/T$. In the same time interval, an individual chosen at random has a probability $b\,\delta t$ of dying. Notice that in assuming a and b are constant, we are assuming there is no change in the age structure of the population with time.

Then
$$\delta x = (a-b)\,x\,\delta t = kx\,\delta t \quad \text{or} \quad dx/dt = kx,$$

i.e.
$$t = \int 1/kx\,dx,$$

$$\therefore \quad \ln x = C + kt, \tag{3.1}$$

or
$$x = A\,e^{kt}.$$

This pattern of growth is often referred to as logarithmic growth, because if $\ln x$ is plotted against t the result is a straight line. There is typically a logarithmic phase in the growth of a bacterial colony, before the supply of nutrients begins to run out and growth to slow down. If we ignore deaths, the generation time $T = 1/a = 1/k$, and k can easily be estimated from equation (3.1).

B. The logistic equation

We will now suppose that the supply of nutrients is sufficient to maintain a steady population of X_E, and that the rate of increase is proportional to $(X_E - x)$, where x is the actual density. So by analogy with equation (2.10), we have

$$dx/dt = C(X_E - x)\,x, \tag{3.2}$$

or
$$t = \int \frac{dx}{C(X_E - x)\,x}.$$

The integral can be evaluated by writing

$$\frac{1}{(X_E - x)\,x} = \frac{R}{x} + \frac{S}{X_E - x},$$

and finding the constants R and S. Thus

$$\frac{1}{(X_E - x)x} = \frac{R(X_E - x) + Sx}{(X_E - x)x}.$$

$$\therefore \quad R(X_E - x) + Sx = 1,$$

$$\therefore \quad RX_E - Rx + Sx = 1$$

so
$$R = S = 1/X_E,$$

and
$$t = \frac{1}{CX_E} \left\{ \int \frac{dx}{x} + \int \frac{dx}{X_E - x} \right\}$$

$$= \frac{1}{CX_E} \left\{ \ln x - \ln |X_E - x| \right\} + B.$$

$$\therefore \quad t = \frac{1}{CX_E} \ln \left| \frac{x}{X_E - x} \right| + B. \tag{3.3}$$

Equation (3.3) gives t, the time taken to reach any particular population density x, in terms of the equilibrium density X_E, the rate of increase when x is small, CX_E, and an arbitrary constant B which can be chosen to fit the initial conditions. Notice that in (3.3), to every value of x there is only one value of t. In other words, (3.3) does not describe an oscillation, in which values of x would recur many times. The form of (3.3) is shown in fig. 13.

Equation (3.2) can be solved exactly, because the integral can be evaluated in terms of a function of x—i.e. $\ln x$—which has been tabulated. Unfortunately many of the differential equations obtained in science cannot be solved in terms of tabulated functions. This is not to say that there is no 'solution'—i.e. that there is no relationship between x and t which would satisfy the equation, but merely that the relationship cannot be expressed in terms of functions which someone has taken the trouble to tabulate.

If an equation cannot be solved in terms of tabulated functions, it is usually possible to find an approximate solution numerically for any particular values of the constants. In the same way, we saw earlier that recurrence relations can easily be solved in particular cases by numerical methods.

The method of solving a simple differential equation by numerical

methods will be illustrated for equation (3.2), so that the solution
can be compared with the analytical solution.

The equation can be written

$$\delta x = C(X_E - x) . x \, \delta t. \tag{3.4}$$

Consider for example a population of *Daphnia* whose density is
adequately described by the logistic equation (in practice, the
logistic equation is usually an inadequate description in such a case,

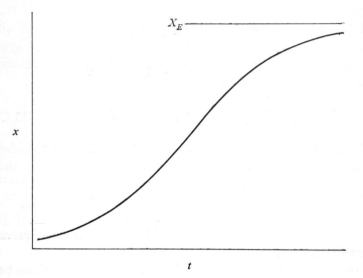

Fig. 13. The logistic equation.

because it ignores the age structure of the population). Let the
equilibrium density $X_E = 10$ per unit area, and let the initial density
be 1 per unit area. Suppose that when the density is low ($x \ll X_E$),
the daily increase in the population is 4 %. Thus if t is measured in
days, when x is small, $\qquad \delta x \simeq C X_E x \, \delta t,$

so that $\qquad \dfrac{\delta x}{x} = 0.04 \delta t = 10C \, \delta t \quad \text{or} \quad C = 0.004,$

and equation (3.4) becomes

$$\delta x = 0.004(X_E - x) x \, \delta t. \tag{3.5}$$

Before using (3.5) to calculate successive values of x, we have to choose a value of the time interval δt. We could choose an interval of 1 day. But clearly the shorter the time interval chosen, the more laborious the calculation. How are we to decide?

In replacing the differential equation by equation (3.5), we are in effect assuming that the slope of the curve between time t and time $t + \delta t$ remains constant, and equal to its true value at time t. Therefore if we are to get a reasonably accurate answer, we must choose δt so that δx does not change too greatly from one time interval to the next.

This condition is satisfied if δt is taken as 1 day. However we will take a much larger interval, $\delta t = 25$ days, and can then see how large the changes in δx are from one interval to the next, and we can also compare the approximate and exact solutions.

Thus for a time interval $\delta t = 25$, we have

$$\delta x = 0 \cdot 1 (X_E - x) x,$$

and so:

t days	0	25	50	75	100	125	150	175
x	1	1·9	3·44	5·70	8·15	9·66	9·99	10
$X_E - x$	9	8·1	6·56	4·30	1·85	0·34	0·01	—
δx		0·9	1·54	2·26	2·45	1·51	0·33	0·01

This arithmetical solution is compared with the exact solution (equation 3.3) in fig. 14. It will be seen that the agreement is reasonably close, even though large differences occur in the value of δx from one interval to the next. The agreement would of course have been better had we taken δt as one day.

Many more refined methods of finding numerical solutions to differential equations have been developed. But it would be out of place to discuss them here, particularly because nowadays if laborious calculations are required to solve an equation, the calculations should be performed by a computer.

It is worth noticing that (3.4) is formally equivalent to (2.10), which could be rewritten

$$X_{n+1} - X_n = \delta X = c(X_E - X_n) X_n. \tag{3.6}$$

Equation (2.10) describes the growth of a population with annual generations, but in deriving both equations it was assumed that the rate of increase is proportional to the difference between the actual and the equilibrium densities. But in (3.6), δX represents the change in density in one year, and may therefore vary greatly from year to year, whereas in (3.4) δt must be chosen so that δx does not change greatly from one year to the next.

A consequence of this difference is that equation (2.10) can lead to oscillations, damped or undamped, whereas (3.4) cannot. This is in line with our earlier conclusion that oscillations are likely to arise from a delay in feedback.

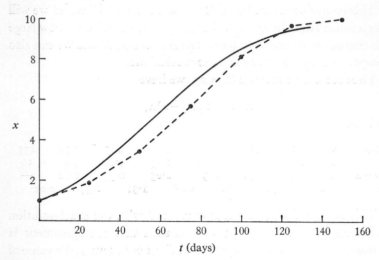

Fig. 14. A comparison of the exact solution of the logistic equation (full line) with an approximate solution obtained by iteration (broken line).

c. Predator–Prey

Equations (2.15) and (2.16) can be rewritten

$$
\left.
\begin{aligned}
x_{n+1} - x_n = \Delta x_n &= -\frac{R-1}{r}x_n - \frac{CX_E}{r}y_n, \\
y_{n+1} - y_n = \Delta y_n &= \frac{(R-1)(r-1)}{CX_E}x_n.
\end{aligned}
\right\}
$$

In these equations, x_n and y_n represent, not the absolute numbers of prey and predators, but the departures of those numbers from their equilibrium values X_s and Y_s. Δx_n and Δy_n represent the changes in x and y between one year and the next—changes which may be large.

A corresponding pair of equations can be obtained for a prey and predator reproducing continuously. Without retracing the argument in detail, it is possible to see that the appropriate equations are

$$\frac{dx}{dt} = -\frac{R-1}{r}x - \frac{CX_E}{r}y \tag{3.7}$$

and

$$\frac{dy}{dt} = \frac{(R-1)(r-1)}{CX_E}x, \tag{3.8}$$

where $X = X_s + x$ = number of prey species,

$\qquad Y = Y_s + y$ = number of predator species,

X_s, Y_s are the equilibrium densities of prey and predator respectively,

X_E is the equilibrium density of the prey in the absence of predators,

R, r are the maximum reproductive rates of the two species, so that $dX/dt = (R-1)X$ when X is small and predators are absent, and

$dY/dt = (r-1)Y$ when $X = X_E$.

The first step in solving equations (3.7) and (3.8) is to eliminate x, as follows:

$$x = \frac{CX_E}{(R-1)(r-1)}\frac{dy}{dt}; \quad \frac{dx}{dt} = \frac{CX_E}{(R-1)(r-1)}\frac{d^2y}{dt^2};$$

and substituting in (3.7) and simplifying gives

$$\frac{d^2y}{dt^2} + \frac{(R-1)}{r}\frac{dy}{dt} + \frac{(R-1)(r-1)}{r}y = 0. \tag{3.9}$$

This equation is of the type solved in appendix 5. Since both $(R-1)$ and $(r-1)$ are positive, the coefficients $(R-1)/r$ and $(R-1)(r-1)/r$ are likewise positive. It is shown in the appendix that if $[(R-1)/r]^2 - 4(R-1)(r-1)/r > 0$, which reduces to $R > (2r-1)^2$, the system is damped; if $R < (2r-1)^2$, there are oscillations whose amplitude decreases with time.

Equation (3.9) cannot give a divergent oscillation if the coefficients are positive. It does not follow that a predator–prey system can give large oscillations only if generations are separate. In equations (3.7) and (3.8) it is assumed that an increase in prey results in an immediate increase in predators. But even for a predator breeding throughout the year, there would be a time lag before the additional offspring grew up and themselves started hunting for prey. This time lag could cause an otherwise damped system to oscillate.

D. Competing species

Equation (3.2) could be rewritten in the form

$$\frac{dx}{dt} = (a - bx)\, x.$$

In this form, the term $-bx$ represents the inhibiting effect one member of a species has on the reproduction of other members of the same species. Suppose now we have two competing species, X and Y, whose density is given by x and y. Competition implies that members of each species have an inhibiting effect on the reproduction of the other. Thus we can write

$$\left.\begin{aligned}
\frac{dx}{dt} &= (a - bx - cy)\, x, \\
\frac{dy}{dt} &= (e - fx - gy)\, y,
\end{aligned}\right\} \tag{3.10}$$

where the term $-cy$ measures the inhibiting effect of species Y on the reproduction of X, and the term $-fx$ the inhibiting effect of X on the reproduction of Y. It is reasonable to say that the species compete if c and f are positive.

The interesting question to be asked about these equations is whether an equilibrium exists when neither x nor y are zero—i.e. can the two species co-exist in the same region? The alternative is that one or other will become extinct. If an equilibrium exists, is it stable? If it is not, then even if the densities of the two species are initially at their equilibrium values, any small departure will lead to the extinction of one species.

The existence of an equilibrium, and its stability, can be investigated graphically.

An equilibrium exists when dx/dt and dy/dt are zero—i.e. when no change takes place in time, i.e.

$$x(a-bx-cy) = 0,$$
$$y(e-fx-gy) = 0.$$

Two equilibrium points are given by

$$x = 0, y = e/g \quad \text{and} \quad y = 0, x = a/b.$$

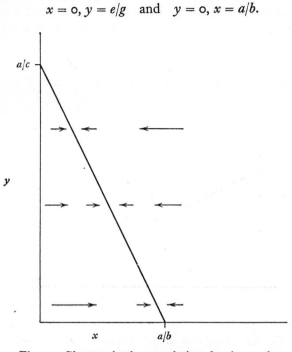

Fig. 15. Changes in the population density x when two species are competing.

These correspond to the equilibrium densities of each species in the absence of the other. A third equilibrium exists when

$$a-bx-cy = 0,$$
$$e-fx-gy = 0.$$

This pair of simultaneous equations can easily be solved algebraically. But since we are also interested in the stability of the equilibrium, it will be more illuminating to solve them graphically.

$a-bx-cy = 0$ represents a straight line, shown in fig. 15.

Any values of the densities x and y of the two populations can be represented as a point on this plane. (Since the densities cannot be negative, the point must lie in the quandrant shown.) For any point above and to the right of the line, the value of $a - bx - cy$ will be negative. Hence, from equation (3.10) dx/dt will be negative, and so x will decrease. For points below and to the left of the line, x will increase. The further from the line a point is, the faster will be the change in x. These conclusions are illustrated by the arrows in fig. 15.

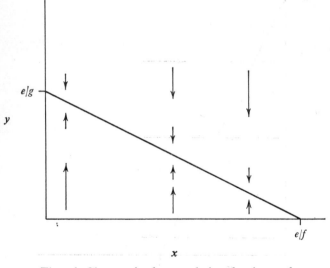

Fig. 16. Changes in the population density y when two species are competing.

Fig. 15 tells us nothing about how y will change with time. This can be deduced from fig. 16.

This figure shows the line $e - fx - gy = 0$.

If we want to know what will happen to the populations starting from any particular values of x and y, we can deduce this by combining the two figures, as in fig. 17. The direction of change has been found by 'adding' the arrows by vector addition, as is done in mechanics when adding forces by use of the 'parallelogram of forces'.

Clearly there is a stable equilibrium at the point of intersection of the two lines. In drawing this figure, however, we have assumed that

$$\frac{a}{c} > \frac{e}{g} \quad \text{and} \quad \frac{a}{b} < \frac{e}{f}. \tag{3.11}$$

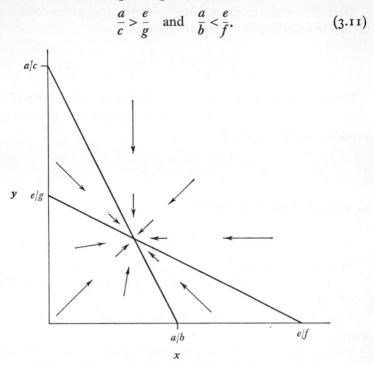

Fig. 17. Changes in the population densities x and y when two species are competing.

The biological significance of these assumptions will be considered in a moment. But first we must consider the consequences of the three possible assumptions:

$$\text{(i)} \quad \frac{a}{c} > \frac{e}{g} \quad \text{and} \quad \frac{a}{b} > \frac{e}{f}.$$

No equilibrium with both species present exists, and species X wins.

$$\text{(ii)} \quad \frac{a}{c} < \frac{e}{g} \quad \text{and} \quad \frac{a}{b} < \frac{e}{f}.$$

Again, no equilibrium with both species present exists, and species Y wins.

$$\text{(iii)} \quad \frac{a}{c} < \frac{e}{g} \quad \text{and} \quad \frac{a}{b} > \frac{e}{f}.$$

An unstable equilibrium exists. The winner in competition depends on the initial densities of the two species.

We will now return to consider the significance of the conditions for stable co-existence of the two species,

$$\frac{a}{c} > \frac{e}{g} \quad \text{and} \quad \frac{a}{b} < \frac{e}{f}.$$

Note that a and e represent the intrinsic rates of increase of the two species when rare. Suppose for simplicity that $a = e$. Then conditions (3.11) reduce to

$$\frac{1}{c} > \frac{1}{g}, \quad \frac{1}{b} < \frac{1}{f};$$

or, since all the constants are positive

$$c < g, \quad b > f.$$

These conditions can be stated verbally:

(i) The inhibiting effect of Y on X is less than that of Y on itself, and

(ii) The inhibiting effect of X on Y is less than that of X on itself.

Thus if for example the species were limited by food, and if their food was in part common and in part species-specific, these conditions would probably be satisfied. But if the two species were micro-organisms each of which released into the surrounding medium a toxic substance which had a greater inhibiting effect on the other species than on itself, then the situation would correspond to (iii) above, i.e. an unstable equilibrium.

E. The effects of age structure

A complete analysis of the behaviour of a population with over-lapping generations would allow for the fact that both fertility and mortality vary, often in a complicated way, with age. Unless fertility and mortality are very simple functions of age, the best that can be done is to solve particular problems by arithmetical methods. The calculations, although not particularly difficult, can be very laborious. But some idea of the effects of age structure can be obtained by considering a simple case.

The case to be considered is that in which there are adult and larval stages which do not complete with one another for food or other resources. We shall further assume that the population is regulated by limiting factors acting on the adults, food and resources for the larvae being present in excess.

Let x_t be the number of adults of all ages alive at time t. We will suppose that the probability that an adult individual will die in a given time interval is constant and independent both of its age and of the population density. Hence the number of adults dying in a time interval δt is $\mu x_t \delta t$, where μ is constant. The assumption that μ is independent of age implies that few individuals live long enough in natural conditions for senescence to bring about an increased probability of dying. There are data suggesting that this is true of many species of birds, but nothing is known of the longevity of insects (to which the present treatment of separate adult and larval stages is more relevant) in nature. The assumption that μ is independent of population density implies that population regulation works on fertility and not on mortality.

We assume that the number of eggs laid by each adult (i.e. half the number laid by each female if there is a 1:1 sex ratio) in interval δt follows the logistic relation, and is equal to $(a - bx_t) \delta t$. This assumes that fertility, like mortality, is independent of age. Let the probability that an egg will survive to become an adult be C, and the time taken from egg to adult be T. Since it was assumed earlier that there are no limiting factors influencing the larval stages, C and T are constants, and not functions of x.

Hence the number of new adults metamorphosing in the interval t to $t + \delta t$ is

$$C(a - bx_{t-T}) x_{t-T} \delta t;$$

i.e. it is C times the number of eggs laid in the time interval $t - T$ to $t - T + \delta t$.

Hence
$$\delta x = C(a - bx_{t-T}) x_{t-T} \delta t - \mu x_t \delta t. \qquad (3.12)$$

This equation can easily be solved numerically for particular values of C, a, b, μ and T.

The equation can be rewritten

$$\delta x = (A - Bx_{t-T}) x_{t-T} \, \delta t - \mu x_t \, \delta t. \qquad (3.13)$$

A is the number of eggs laid per adult in unit time which in optimal conditions (low x) survive to become adults. For numerical calculations, we will choose a time scale such that when $\delta t = 1$, A is $\frac{1}{4}$; this should ensure δx is small compared with x, which is necessary if our numerical solution is to approximate the true solution. We will assume that during this time interval the probability that an adult will die is $1/20$, and that the time taken for an egg to develop into an adult is 30 intervals.

Thus
$$A = 0.25, \quad T = 30, \quad k = 0.05,$$

and hence
$$\delta x = (0.25 - Bx_{t-30}) x_{t-30} - 0.05 x_t.$$

The value of B is determined from the equilibrium density, X_E. Thus at equilibrium $\delta x = 0$, and

$$x_{t-30} = x_t = X_E,$$

and hence
$$(0.25 - BX_E) X_E - 0.05 X_E = 0,$$

hence
$$X_E = 0 \quad \text{or} \quad \frac{0.20}{B}.$$

Thus if we choose as a unit area one which at equilibrium will support 10 adults, $B = 0.02$.

Thus
$$\delta x = (0.25 - 0.02 x_{t-30}) x_{t-30} - 0.05 x_t. \qquad (3.14)$$

We will investigate numerically a case in which a number of adult animals equal to half the equilibrium number are suddenly introduced into the habitat. Thus at time $t = 0$, $x_0 = 5$, and for the first 30 time intervals, $x_{t-30} = 0$.

For these first 30 intervals, there is a logarithmic decrease,

$$\delta x = -0.05 x_t \quad \text{or} \quad x_{t+1} = 0.95 x_t,$$

and hence

$t =$	0	1	2	...	29	30
$x_t =$	5	4.75	4.51	...	1.095	1.040

Subsequently, the behaviour of the population can be calculated as follows:

t	30	31	32	33
x_t	1·04	1·738	2·388	2·991
x_{t-30}	5	4·75	4·51	—
$0·02x_{t-30}$	0·100	0·095	0·090	—
$0·25 - 0·02x_{t-30}$	0·150	0·155	0·160	—
$[0·25 - 0·02x_{t-30}]x_{t-30}$	0·750	0·737	0·722	—
$0·05x_t$	0·052	0·087	0·119	—
δx	0·698	0·650	0·603	—

The results of such a computation are shown in fig. 18.

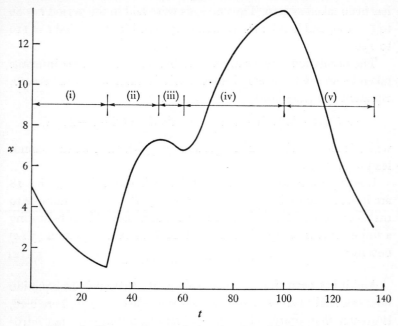

Fig. 18. Changes in population density with time for the imaginary example considered in the text.

It is apparent that the population shows oscillatory behaviour. The details of the oscillation are as follows:

Period (i) $t = 0$ to $t = 30$. Deaths, but no recruitment.

Period (ii) $t = 30$ to $t = 50$. Increase in population, as the eggs laid during period (i) metamorphose into adults.

Period (iii) $t = 50$ to 60. Slight decrease, because the adult population from $t = 20$ to 30 was very small, and hence few eggs were laid which would hatch during this period.

Period (iv) $t = 60$ to $t = 100$. Renewed increase as the number of new adults increases.

Period (v) $t = 100$ to $t = 140$. Decrease in numbers. Not many new adults emerge, because in the period $t = 70$ to $t = 110$ the adult population was above its equilibrium level, and therefore few eggs were laid. Note that $A - Bx$, the number of eggs laid per adult per unit time, is negative when x is greater than 12·5. Clearly an animal cannot lay a negative number of eggs, and so when $x > 12·5$, $A - Bx$ has been taken as zero. Thus no eggs were laid in the period $t = 86$ to $t = 106$, and hence no new adults emerged in the period $t = 116$ to 136.

The oscillations are clearly due to the delay of 30 time intervals taken by an egg to develop into an adult. Thus if we take T as zero, equation (3.13) becomes

$$\delta x = (A - Bx)\,x\,\delta t - \mu x\,\delta t \quad \text{or} \quad dx/dt = (A - \mu - Bx)\,x,$$

which is identical in form to equation (3.2), which as we saw cannot lead to an oscillation.

It is important to make sure that the oscillations shown in fig. 18 are indeed due to the delay represented by $T = 30$, and not due to the fact that the differential equation has been solved by substituting a finite difference equation. If we take T as zero, equation (3.14) becomes

$$\delta x = (0·20 - 0·02x)\,x,$$

And it has been shown earlier (see p. 26) that such an equation does not lead to an oscillation unless the constant term, here 0·20, is greater than unity. Thus the oscillations found were not introduced by the approximate method of solution. This justifies our choice of a time interval giving $A = 0·25$.

An oscillation of an experimental population in a situation very approximately corresponding to that considered above is shown in fig. 19.

This example of the effects of age structure on the behaviour of a population has been chosen for its simplicity. In general, both the fertility and the mortality of individuals is likely to be a function of their age, and of the population density at the time—and perhaps of many other factors as well. To predict the behaviour of such a population requires that the effects of age, density, and other relevant factors on fertility and mortality be known. To calculate the future behaviour of a population is then laborious but not in principle difficult. The method resembles that used above, except that instead of calculating for each time interval a single measure, x,

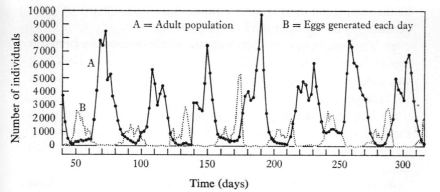

Fig. 19. Numbers of the blowfly *Lucilia* in a population cage. Larvae received unlimited food, and adults received a limited supply of 0·5 gm. of liver daily. Full line, adult population; broken line, eggs laid per day. (After Nicholson, A. J. (1954). *Aust. J. Zool.* **2**, 9.)

of adult population density, it is necessary to calculate a number of separate measures, $(x_0)_t$, $(x_1)_t$, $(x_2)_t$ ... corresponding to the number of adults in different age classes alive at a given time. It is rare for sufficient information to be available to make such calculations worth while. The real value of the calculations which led to fig. 18, and indeed of most of the calculations in this and the preceding chapter, is in giving an approximate picture of the effects of various factors on the behaviour of populations. The picture may be approximate, but it is better than could be achieved by a purely verbal argument.

Examples

1   A logarithmically growing culture of bacteria increases from 2×10^6 cells to 3×10^8 cells in 5 hours. What is the time between successive fissions if (a) there is no mortality; (b) 10 % of cells originating from one fission die before the next?

2   A bacterial population grows according to the logistic equation, with an equilibrium density of 5×10^8 cells per ml. When the population density is low, it doubles every 40 minutes. What will be the population density after 2 hours if initially it is (a) 10^8 cells per ml.; (b) 10^9 cells per ml.?

3   The time in minutes between successive fissions in a bacterial culture is $40 + 10^{-7}x$, where x is the density in cells per ml. How long will it take for the density to increase from 10^8 cells per ml. to 10^9 cells per ml.?

4   In a *Drosophila* population cage, food is supplied in excess for the adults, but in limited amounts for the larvae. Adult females lay 10 eggs a day. The sex ratio is 1 : 1. 10 % of all living adults die each day.

An egg hatches into a larva 24 hours after being laid. 4 days after hatching the larva pupates, and 5 days after pupation an adult emerges. There is mortality only in the larval stage of development. The probability that a particular egg will survive to pupate is $(1 + x/100)^{-1}$, where x is the number of eggs laid during the four previous days; i.e. it is the number of larvae there would be in the cage when the egg in question hatches, if mortality were ignored.

(a) What is the equilibrium density of adults in the cage?

What would be the equilibrium density if:

(b) the number of eggs laid daily per female were doubled?

(c) the daily adult mortality were halved?

(d) half the adults emerging each day were removed from the cage?

If a cage were started by introducing 200 adults, how, approximately, would the number of adults vary during the next 30 days?

A. The concepts of probability and independence

The main mathematical concept needed in genetics is that of probability. When we speak of the 'probability' of an event, we mean the frequency with which that event occurs in a long sequence of trials. Thus the probability that a six will turn up in a single throw of a six-sided die is approximately 1/6. For most dice it is not exactly 1/6, because the spots are marked with small depressions on the surface, so that the six face is lighter than the others and so finishes uppermost more often. The important points then are:

(i) The probability of an event is defined as the frequency with which it occurs in a long sequence of trials: i.e. it is the number of 'successes' (e.g. sixes) divided by the total number of 'trials' (e.g. throws). A probability is therefore a number lying between 0 (the event never happens) and 1 (the event always happens).

(ii) All statements of probability rest ultimately on empirical measurements. Thus we know that the probability of a six is 1/6, not merely because a die has six sides, but because such dice have been thrown a large number of times, and the six falls upper-most on about 1/6 of the throws.

To take a genetical example, it is approximately true that the probability that baby born in this country will be a boy is one half. Actually the fraction of all babies born that are boys varies somewhat. In England and Wales at the present time approximately 106 boys are born for every 100 girls; but to simplify the argument the proportion of boys will be taken to be exactly one half.

We can then ask the question: what is the probability that a family consisting of two children will consist of two boys? A simple but erroneous argument is as follows: there are three possible kinds of family—two boys, two girls, and one boy and one girl—so the probability of two boys is one third. The argument is false because families of one boy and one girl are more probable (i.e. occur more frequently) than the other two kinds of family.

There are two lines of argument which lead to the correct conclusion. The first is to argue that when birth order is taken into account, there are four kinds of family and not three—boy boy, boy girl, girl boy and girl girl. If we assume that these four are equally frequent, the probability of two boys is one quarter. Observation shows this answer to be correct, but why was it correct to assume that these four kinds of family are equally frequent?

The assumption that has been made becomes a little clearer if we express the argument in a different form, as follows. In one half of all families of two, the older child is a boy; and in one half of these, the second child is also a boy. Hence the probability of two boys is $\frac{1}{2} \times \frac{1}{2} = \frac{1}{4}$. Similarly, the probability of each of the other kinds of family is $\frac{1}{4}$. In this argument, we have not only assumed that half of all births are boys, but also that this remains true of the second child when it is known that the first child was a boy. In other words, we have assumed that the sex of the second child is *independent* of that of the first.

The concept of independence is important. It is defined as follows. Let there be two events, A and B, with probabilities $P(A)$ and $P(B)$. The events are independent if the probability that both occur, $P(A \text{ and } B)$, is equal to $P(A) \times P(B)$. In other words, two events are independent if the frequency with which both events occur is equal to the product of the frequencies of the two events taken singly. In the example, event A is that the older child is a boy, and event B that the younger child is a boy; we assumed that the probability that both are boys is equal to $P(A) \times P(B)$.

The grounds for assuming that two events are independent are ultimately empirical. Thus if one quarter of all families of two children in fact consist of two boys, we can take this as evidence that the sexes of the first and second child are independent. Actually there are slightly more families of two boys than would be expected from the frequency of male births. There are many possible reasons for this; for example, some women may provide a uterine environment more favourable to the survival of male foetuses, others of female foetuses. But the effect is a small one, and in what follows I shall assume that the sexes of successive births are independent.

To summarise:

(i) The probability of an event is the frequency with which it occurs in a long sequence of trials. If two events are mutually exclusive and the only ones possible (e.g. head and tail in a single toss, or boy and girl in a single birth), and their probabilities are p and q respectively, then $p + q = 1$.

(ii) Two events are said to be independent if the probability that both occur (e.g. that in two tosses of a die, both are sixes) is equal to the product of the probabilities of the two events taken separately (i.e. $1/6 \times 1/6 = 1/36$).

(iii) Statements about the probabilities and about the independence of events rest ultimately on empirical evidence.

B. The binomial theorem

Assuming that the sex ratio is $1:1$ and that the sexes of successive children are independent, we can ask what is the probability, in a family of three children, of 1 boy and 2 girls. It is fairly easy to see the answer to this question, but as an introduction to more difficult questions it is worth taking it slowly.

We first ask what is the probability of a particular kind of family, taking into account birth order, with 1 boy and 2 girls—for example boy girl girl. The answer is clearly $\frac{1}{2} \times \frac{1}{2} \times \frac{1}{2} = \frac{1}{8}$.

Next we ask how many kinds of families there are with 1 boy and 2 girls. The answer is three—boy girl girl, girl boy girl and girl girl boy. Hence the probability of a family with 1 boy and 2 girls is $3 \times \frac{1}{8} = \frac{3}{8}$.

This is an example of a theorem known as the binomial theorem. Before stating this in its general form, a more difficult example will be given. If an albino and a coloured mouse are crossed, the F_1 (i.e. the first generation offspring) are coloured, and in the F_2 (i.e. the second generation obtained by mating together two individuals from the F_1) we 'expect' 3 coloured to 1 white. By 'expect', we mean that if we count a large number of offspring from such crosses, one quarter will be white. Suppose we have a single litter of 5 F_2 mice;

what is the probability that it will consist of 3 coloured and 2 white mice?

As before, we calculate first the probability of a particular litter, allowing for birth order; for example, a litter in which the first two mice born were white and the last three coloured, represented as follows:

birth position	1	2	3	4	5
colour	○	○	●	●	●

The probability that the first two mice will be white is $\frac{1}{4} \times \frac{1}{4}$, and that the last three will be coloured is $\frac{3}{4} \times \frac{3}{4} \times \frac{3}{4}$. Hence the probability of this particular litter is $(\frac{1}{4})^2 (\frac{3}{4})^3$.

We now want to know how many kinds of litter there are with two white mice, allowing for birth order. This is equivalent to asking 'In how many ways can I select two birth positions, corresponding to the two white mice, out of five?' The first position can be selected in 5 ways, and once this has been done, there are 4 ways in which the second position can be selected. This might suggest that there are $5 \times 4 = 20$ kinds of litter, but this is a mistake. In the twenty litters, we would count the litter represented above twice; we would count a litter in which the first birth position was selected first and the second birth position was selected second, and also a litter in which the second position was selected first and the first position was selected second. The same is true for all other kinds of litter—for example, ○ ● ● ● ○. Thus the number of distinguishable kinds of litter is $\frac{1}{2}(5 \times 4) = 10$. You should satisfy yourself of the truth of this statement by listing the ten possible litters.

Hence the probability of a litter with 2 white and 3 coloured mice is

$$10 \times (\tfrac{1}{4})^2 \times (\tfrac{3}{4})^3 = \tfrac{135}{512}.$$

Notice that the answer could be written

$$\frac{5!}{2!\,3!}(\tfrac{1}{4})^2 (\tfrac{3}{4})^3,$$

where 5! denotes $5 \times 4 \times 3 \times 2 \times 1$, and is read as '5 factorial'. This suggests the following general theorem: If in each of

n independent trials, the probability of a success is p, then the probability of r successes is

$$\frac{n!}{r!(n-r)!}p^r(1-p)^{n-r}.$$

If, as is customary, we write $1-p = q$, we can reformulate this theorem as follows:

If in each of n independent trials the probability of a success is p, the probabilities of $0, 1, 2, \ldots, r, \ldots, n$ successes are given by successive terms of the expansion of $(q+p)^n \ldots$ i.e. by

$$q^n, \quad nq^{n-1}p, \quad \frac{n(n-1)}{2}q^{n-2}p^2, \cdots \frac{n!}{r!(n-r)!}q^{n-r}p^r, \cdots p^n.$$

No formal proof of this theorem will be given. The proof resembles that given in the particular case just considered. Thus the probability that the first r trials out of n are successes and the rest failures is $p^r(1-p)^{n-r}$, and the number of ways of choosing r objects (i.e. successful trials) out of n (total trials) is $\dfrac{n!}{r!(n-r)!}$.

This 'binomial theorem' can be used to calculate the probability of any particular family from known parents. There is one additional trick which is often useful in calculating probabilities. Suppose for example that we want to know the probability that, in a litter of $8\,F_2$ mice from a cross of an albino to a coloured mouse, there will be at least one white mouse. It would be very laborious to calculate the probabilities that there will be $1, 2, 3 \ldots$ up to 8 white mice, and add these probabilities together. Fortunately there is no need. We calculate the probability that there will be no white mice, i.e.

$$P(0) = (\tfrac{3}{4})^8 \simeq 0.1001.$$

Then the probability that there is at least one white mouse follows directly, because

$$P \text{ (at least 1)} = 1 - P(0) \simeq 0.8999.$$

In other words, when it is laborious to calculate the probability that something will happen, try calculating the probability that it won't.

c. Conditional probability

So far we have considered only events which are independent. But we often want to know the probability that two events will occur, when the probability of one of them depends on whether the other has or has not occurred.

What for example is the probability that two cards drawn at random from a pack are both spades? The probability that the first card drawn is a spade is $13/52 = \frac{1}{4}$. Once a spade has been drawn, there are 51 cards left in the pack, of which 12 are spades. Hence the probability that the second card is a spade, given that the first one is, is $12/51$ and not $\frac{1}{4}$. Hence the probability that both are spades is $\frac{1}{4} \times 12/51 = 1/17$. (At this point, you should ponder the fact that the same conclusion would follow if both cards were drawn simultaneously).

This class of problem arises in contexts other than gambling. Suppose for example we want to know the probability that a girl who is a member of a family of three children has an older brother. Obviously this will depend on whether the girl is the first, second or third child in the family. To solve the problem, it will help to be clear what we mean by probability in this case. A probability refers to the frequency of 'successes' to 'trials'. In this case, we might imagine ourselves collecting all the girls in this country, and asking each one whether she belonged to a family of three children. Those who answered yes would constitute our population of 'trials'. Each of these would then be asked whether she had an older brother; those answering yes a second time would be 'successes'.

Of girls belonging to families of three children:

$\frac{1}{3}$ would be the first child, and of these none would have an older brother;

$\frac{1}{3}$ would be the second child, and of these half would have an older brother;

$\frac{1}{3}$ would be the third child, and of these $\frac{3}{4}$ would have an older brother ($1 - \frac{1}{4} = \frac{3}{4}$ is the probability that, of two older sibs, at least one is a boy).

Thus the required probability is

$$\tfrac{1}{3} \times 0 + \tfrac{1}{3} \times \tfrac{1}{2} + \tfrac{1}{3} \times \tfrac{3}{4} = 5/12.$$

The procedure adopted here is made easier in complex cases by introducing a new notation. We write

$P(A)$ = The probability (P) that A happens.

$P(A|H)$ = The probability that A happens, given that H is the case.

Then if H_1, H_2 and H_3 are three states of affairs of which one and only one is the case (H_1, H_2 and H_3 are then said to be 'mutually exclusive and the only possible'), then

$$P(A) = P(A|H_1) \times P(H_1) + P(A|H_2) \times P(H_2) + P(A|H_3) \times P(H_3).$$

$$(4.1)$$

No formal proof of this theorem will be given. It is merely a shorthand way of writing the procedure adopted for the problem of the girl and her elder brother, with A meaning 'the girl has an elder brother', and H_1, H_2 and H_3 meaning that the girl is, respectively, the first, second and third child out of three. The method can be applied for any finite number of possible conditions $H_1, H_2, ..., H_n$.

H_1, H_2, etc., are sometimes referred to as 'hypotheses', but the term is unfortunate, since it suggests that they resemble a universal hypothesis such as Avogadro's hypothesis. If they did, it would be absurd to write $P(H_1)$, etc., since one cannot sensibly speak of the frequency with which Avogadro's hypothesis is the case. In the example considered, H_1, etc., refer to particular states of affairs which are true in a certain proportion of cases.

The main utility of (4.1) will emerge in the next chapter, but a few examples will be given here. Returning to the F_2 between an albino and a coloured mouse, suppose that a single coloured F_2 mouse, whom we will call Minnie, is crossed to an albino, and a litter of 5 obtained. What is the probability that all five are coloured?

Clearly this will depend on whether Minnie is homozygous coloured (CC) or heterozygous for the albino gene (Cc). In the former case all her offspring will be coloured; in the latter, we expect 1 coloured to 1 albino. Thus we can write P(all 5 coloured) = P (all 5 coloured|Minnie is CC) $\times$ P (Minnie is CC) + P (all 5 coloured| Minnie is Cc) $\times$ P (Minnie is Cc) = $1 \times \frac{1}{3} + (\frac{1}{2})^5 \times \frac{2}{3} = 17/48$.

Now consider a more difficult example. Suppose that in man blue eyes are recessive to brown—i.e. that *BB* and *Bb* have brown eyes and *bb* have blue eyes (this is only approximately true). Suppose also that in a particular human population 36 % of people have blue eyes, 16 % are homozygous for brown eyes, and 48 % are heterozygous. Given that a man has blue eyes and has a brother, what is the probability that the brother's eyes are also blue?

Clearly this depends on whether the man's parents were, for example, both *bb*, in which case the brother is certain to have blue eyes, or were for example both *Bb*, in which case the brother may well have brown eyes.

The first step is to set out a table, giving the different kinds of marriage, with their frequencies, and the proportion of blue-eyed children, as follows:

Father		Mother	Frequency of marriage f	Proportion of blue-eyed children in family p	Relative proportions of blue-eyed children in population $n = f \times p$
BB	×	*BB*	0.16×0.16	0	0
BB *bb*	× ×	*bb* } *BB* }	$2 \times 0.16 \times 0.36$	0	0
BB *Bb*	× ×	*Bb* } *BB* }	$2 \times 0.16 \times 0.48$	0	0
Bb	×	*Bb*	0.48×0.48	$\frac{1}{4}$	0.0576
Bb *bb*	× ×	*bb* } *Bb* }	$2 \times 0.48 \times 0.36$	$\frac{1}{2}$	0.1728
bb	×	*bb*	0.36×0.36	1	0.1296
				Total	0.3600

In writing down the frequencies of different kinds of marriages, we have assumed that the genotypes of husband and wife are independent as far as eye colour is concerned. This would not be the case if, for example, blue-eyed people tend to marry one another. But some assumption has to be made if the original question is to be answered.

It is easy to make mistakes when writing down tables of this kind; fortunately a number of checks are available. First, since there are

3 kinds of parent there are 9 kinds of marriage, and we have listed them all. Second, we should verify that the sum of the entries in the f column is unity. (A final check is provided by the fact that the frequency of blue-eyed children, 0·3600, equals the frequency of blue-eyed parents. But this is only the case, as will emerge in the next chapter, because we have assumed 'random mating', and have chosen frequencies for the parental genotypes which fit the 'Hardy–Weinberg' ratio.)

It follows from the table that of all blue-eyed children, a fraction $\frac{0·0576}{0·3600}$ have two brown-eyed parents, $\frac{0·1728}{0·3600}$ have one brown-eyed parent, and $\frac{0·1296}{0·3600}$ have two blue-eyed parents.

We are now in a position to use (4.1) to calculate the probability, P, that if a blue-eyed man has a brother, the brother will also have blue eyes:

$$P = \frac{0·0576}{0·3600} \times \tfrac{1}{4} + \frac{0·1728}{0·3600} \times \tfrac{1}{2} + \frac{0·1296}{0·3600} \times 1 = 0·64.$$

A reason why one might wish to find such a probability will emerge later, when discussing twin diagnosis.

D. Inverse probability

Calculations of probability start by assuming the truth of some general propositions (e.g. that half the babies born are boys, and that the sexes of successive babies are independent) and calculating the probability (i.e. frequency) of some particular event (e.g. families of 2 boys and 2 girls). The problem of inverse probability is to start from the fact that a particular event or group of events takes place, and to calculate the probability that some general proposition is true. So formulated, the problem is clearly insoluble, and indeed is meaningless if by 'probability' we mean 'frequency of occurrence'. General propositions cannot be true in a certain proportion of cases.

Thus suppose for example we use the genes *vestigial* and *aristapedia* in *Drosophila* in an experiment intended to test Mendel's law of independent assortment, and obtain in the F_2 numbers closely agreeing with the 'expected' 9:3:3:1 ratio. We cannot then ascribe a numerical value to the probability that Mendel's law is true, because a probability is a measure of frequency, and Mendel's law is not sometimes true of *vestigial* and *aristapedia* and sometimes false.

What we can do is calculate the probability of getting this observed result if Mendel's law is true. We can go further, and calculate, again assuming Mendel's law is true, the probability of obtaining a result whose fit with the expected ratio is as bad as or worse than the one we actually obtained—this is what is usually calculated in statistical 'significance tests'. But there is a class of problems in which we adopt a kind of inverse argument to calculate the probability that some proposition is true. The proposition must not be a general one, but one which is sometimes true and sometimes false. An example will make the method clear.

Suppose that a woman of blood group O marries an AB man, and has a pair of boy twins of blood group B. If this is all we know, what is the probability that the twins are monovular—i.e. from a single egg?

Our difficulty is this: if we knew that a pair of twins from such a marriage were monovular, it would be easy to calculate the probability that both had the B blood group; but we have been asked to solve the inverse problem. However, let us do the easy part first. The genetics of the situation is as follows:

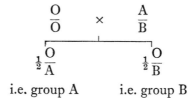

i.e. group A   i.e. group B

Thus for binovular twins, the probability of two B children is $\frac{1}{2} \times \frac{1}{2} = \frac{1}{4}$. For monovular twins, the probability that the first born is B is $\frac{1}{2}$; if he is, the second is sure to be. Hence the probability of two B twins is $\frac{1}{2}$.

Using the notation introduced on page 63, we will write these conclusions as follows:

$$P(2\text{B}|\text{bin}) = \tfrac{1}{4}; \quad P(2\text{B}|\text{mon}) = \tfrac{1}{2}.$$

What we want to know is $P(\text{mon}|2\text{B})$—i.e. the probability that the twins are monovular if both are B. This problem we can only solve if we have some *a priori* knowledge of the frequency of monovular and binovular twins, knowing only that they are of the same sex.

This we can deduce from the observation that 32 % of all twin pairs are of unlike sex (the proportion varies from population to population). These 32 % are necessarily all binovular, and since equal numbers of binovular pairs will be of like and of unlike sex, a further 32 % of twin pairs must be binovular pairs of like sex, giving 64 % of binovular pairs in all. This leaves 36 % of monovular pairs. The argument is illustrated in fig. 20.

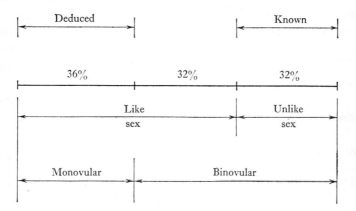

Fig. 20. Method of estimating the frequency of monovular twins.

It follows that of all like-sex twins, a fraction 0·36/0·68 are monovular, and 0·32/0·68 are binovular.

Hence, if we were to collect all the pairs of boy twins from marriages of O ♀ × AB♂ we would find

$$\frac{0\cdot32}{0\cdot68} \times \tfrac{1}{4} \quad \text{are binovular, and both B,}$$

and
$$\frac{0\cdot36}{0\cdot68} \times \tfrac{1}{2} \quad \text{are monovular, and both B.}$$

Hence, the probability that a pair of boy twins are monovular, given that they are both B, is

$$P(\text{mon}|2\text{B}) = \frac{0 \cdot 36}{0 \cdot 68} \times \frac{1}{2} \div \left(\frac{0 \cdot 36}{0 \cdot 68} \times \frac{1}{2} + \frac{0 \cdot 32}{0 \cdot 68} \times \frac{1}{4}\right) = \frac{9}{13}.$$

This is the solution to our problem. Notice that if we had written the *a priori* probabilities that a like-sex twin pair are monovular and binovular as $P(\text{mon})$ and $P(\text{bin})$ respectively, our solution has the form

$$P(\text{mon}|2\text{B}) = \frac{P(2\text{B}|\text{mon}) \times P(\text{mon})}{P(2\text{B}|\text{mon}) \times P(\text{mon}) + P(2\text{B}|\text{bin}) \times P(\text{bin})}.$$

This is a special case of Bayes' theorem. Thus suppose H_1 and H_2 are propositions of which one and only one is true, and B is some result whose probability depends on which proposition is true. The probability that both H_1 and B are true can be written $P(H_1 + B)$.

Then

$$P(H_1 + B) = P(H_1)\,P(B|H_1)$$

and similarly

$$P(H_1 + B) = P(B)\,P(H_1|B).$$

Hence

$$P(H_1|B) = \frac{P(B|H_1)\,P(H_1)}{P(B)}$$

and

$$P(B) = P(B|H_1)\,P(H_1) + P(B|H_2)\,P(H_2)$$

and so

$$P(H_1|B) = \frac{P(B|H_1)\,P(H_1)}{P(B|H_1)\,P(H_1) + P(B|H_2)\,P(H_2)} \qquad (4.2)$$

which is Bayes' Theorem. The theorem can be extended to cases where three or more alternative *a priori* propositions exist. The theorem can be used to calculate the *a posteriori* probability of some proposition H_1, in the light of additional evidence B, provided that

(i) *a priori* probabilities of H_1 and not-H_1, in the absence of knowledge about B, are known.

(ii) the probability of B, given that H_1 or not-H_1 is the case, can be calculated.

The first point is crucial; in the examples considered, the frequency of monovular pairs among like-sexed twins was known.

The theorem can be applied to twin diagnosis even if the geno-types of the parents are not known, provided that the frequencies of genotypes in the population are known and that random mating can be assumed. For example, what is the probability that two blue-eyed boy twins are monovular? With the usual notation

$$P(\text{mon}|2b) = \frac{P(2b|\text{mon})\,P(\text{mon})}{P(2b|\text{mon})\,P(\text{mon}) + P(2b|\text{bin})\,P(\text{bin})}.$$

Now, if we assume the same genotype frequencies as on page 64, 36 % of people have blue eyes.

Hence $P(2b|\text{mon}) = 0.36$.

We have already calculated that for a pair of brothers, and hence for a pair of binovular twins, if one has blue eyes, there is a probability of 0.64 that the other has. Hence

$$P(2b|\text{bin}) = 0.36 \times 0.64.$$

And assuming as before that

$$P(\text{mon}) = 0.36/0.68 \quad \text{and} \quad P(\text{bin}) = 0.32/0.68,$$

we have

$$P(\text{mon}|2b) = 0.36 \times \frac{0.36}{0.68} \div \left(0.36 \times \frac{0.36}{0.68} + 0.36 \times 0.64 \times \frac{0.32}{0.68}\right)$$
$$= 0.638.$$

Before it was known that both twins were blue-eyed, the probability that they were monovular was $0.36/0.68 = 0.530$; the additional evidence has raised the probability to 0.638.

Examples

1 Two unbiased dice are thrown. What is the probability that the numbers showing (a) add up to 9; (b) differ by 2; (c) are different?

2 A red and a green die are thrown. What is the probability that

(a) the number on the red die is even and the number on the green die is less than 3;

(b) the number on the red die is less than three or the number on the green die is more than three;

(c) the number on the red die is 5 given that the sum of the spots on the two dice is 9 or more?

3 5 cards are drawn from a normal pack of 52. What is the probability that (a) they are all the same suit; (b) they include 4 aces?

4 Albinism in mice is due to a recessive gene. An albino is crossed to a pure-bred coloured mouse, and a second generation (F_2) litter of 4 mice is obtained (expectation, 3 coloured : 1 albino). What is the probability that the litter will contain

(a) 3 coloured and 1 albino;

(b) at least 1 albino;

(c) 1 albino, 2 heterozygous coloured, 1 pure-bred coloured;

(d) 2 albino females and 2 coloured males?

5 What proportion of girls from families of 4 children have at least two older brothers?

6 (a) A coloured mouse called Minnie from an F_2 litter similar to that described in question 4 is crossed to an albino male. She has a litter of 5. What is the probability that at least one of them is an albino?

(b) In fact, Minne's litter consists of 5 coloured mice. What is the probability that Minnie carries an albino gene?

7 Of three prisoners, Matthew, Mark and Luke, two are to be executed, but Matthew does not know which. He therefore asks the jailer 'Since either Mark or Luke are certainly going to be executed, you will give me no information about my own chances if you give me the name of one man, either Mark or Luke, who is going to be executed.' Accepting this argument, the jailer truthfully replied 'Mark will be executed'. Thereupon, Matthew felt happier, because before the jailer replied his own chances of execution were 2/3, but afterwards there are only two people, himself and Luke, who could be the one not to be executed, and so his chance of execution is only $\frac{1}{2}$.

Is Matthew right to feel happier?

(This should be called the Serbelloni problem since it nearly wrecked a conference on theoretical biology at the villa Serbelloni in the summer of 1966; it yields at once to common sense or to Bayes' theorem.)

5 THE GENETICS OF POPULATIONS

The fundamental idea of population genetics is that of a 'gene frequency'. Consider a population of diploid organisms, and suppose that at a particular locus there are two, and only two alleles, A and a, present in the population. Then there are three possible genotypes present in the population, AA, Aa and aa. In principle it would be possible to count these genotypes and find their proportions, $P\,AA:Q\,Aa:R\,aa$, where $P+Q+R = 1$. (In practice, it is usually difficult to distinguish the heterozygote Aa from one of the homozygotes AA or aa.) P, Q and R are then the genotype frequencies. From them we can calculate the gene frequencies $p\,A:q\,a$ as follows:

$$p = P+\tfrac{1}{2}Q; \quad q = \tfrac{1}{2}Q+R. \tag{5.1}$$

In so doing, we have 'counted' the A and a genes in the population, by allowing two A genes in an AA homozygote, two a genes in an aa homozygote, and one A and one a gene in an Aa heterozygote.

A. The Hardy–Weinberg ratio

The relations (5.1) hold for all 'autosomal' (i.e. not sex-linked) loci in a diploid, whatever the mating system. The relations enable us to calculate p and q if we know P, Q and R. Thus if a population consists of 60 % AA, 10 % Aa, and 30 % aa, then $p = 0.65$ and $q = 0.35$. But the reverse is not true; we cannot calculate P, Q and R merely from a knowledge of p and q.

It is however possible to find P, Q and R from p and q if we assume 'random mating'; that is, if we assume that the probability that an individual will mate with an AA, Aa or aa partner is independent of the genotype of the individual. Thus, if the frequences of genes A and a are p and q respectively, the probability that a child will inherit gene A from its father is p. The probability that a child will inherit gene A from its mother is likewise p, and, if mating is random, is independent of whether the child also inherited gene A from its father.

Hence the probability that a child inherits gene A from both parents is p^2, and this is equal to P, the frequency of the AA genotype in the population.

This argument can be extended in a tabular form:

gene from father	gene from mother	genotype	frequency
A	A	AA	p^2
A	a	Aa	pq
a	A	Aa	pq
a	a	aa	q^2

Hence the 'Hardy–Weinberg' ratio, which states that if in a diploid population two allelic genes are present in the frequencies $p\,A:q\,a$, then random mating will give rise to zygotes with genotypes in the proportions $p^2\,AA:2pq\,Aa:q^2\,aa$. This ratio is reached in a single generation of random mating, whatever the genotype frequencies in the parental population.

The Hardy–Weinberg ratio is widely assumed to be true in population genetics. The assumption is justified only if mating is random for the genotypes concerned. How are we to decide whether mating is random? In general we cannot. But if we can identify all three genotypes in a sample of a population, we can count them and see whether they agree with the Hardy–Weinberg ratio. If they do, this confirms that mating is random. For example, mating has been shown to be near enough random in this way for blood groups in man, and for black, ginger and tortoise-shell in London's cats. On the other hand, it is known that tall people tend to marry one another, and likewise short people, so mating is not random for genes affecting height. Finally, if we count genotypes in an adult population and find that they depart significantly from the Hardy–Weinberg ratio, this does not prove that mating is non-random; the discrepancy could equally well be caused by differential mortality.

B. Selection

Suppose that in a random-mating population there are two allelic genes A and a, A being dominant to a, and that the probabilities of survival from fertilised egg to breeding adult are:

$$\text{for } AA \text{ and } Aa, \qquad S$$
$$\text{and for } aa, \qquad S(1-k).$$

Thus if k is positive, aa has a lower 'fitness' than AA or Aa. It is assumed that the fertilities of the three genotypes are the same. What will happen to such a population, and how rapidly will it happen? For simplicity, we will assume that generations are separate. The procedure is then to calculate the gene frequency in one generation in terms of the gene frequency at the same stage of the preceding one.

Let the frequency of A in the adults of the nth generation be p_n. Then with random mating, zygotes of the $(n+1)$th generation will be formed with the frequencies.

$$p_n^2 AA : 2p_n(1-p_n)Aa : (1-p_n)^2 aa.$$

The adults of the $(n+1)$th generation will then be in the relative proportions:

$$Sp_n^2 AA : 2Sp_n(1-p_n)Aa : S(1-p_n)^2(1-k)aa. \qquad (5.2)$$

And p_{n+1}, the frequency of A genes in the adults of the $(n+1)$th generation, could then be found by 'counting' the A genes as a fraction of all genes in (5.2). However, this procedure leads to a rather clumsy expression for p_{n+1} in terms of p_n. It turns out that we get a neater expression if we work with $u_n = p_n/(1-p_n)$; i.e. the ratio of A genes to a genes in the nth generation.

Thus if we divide each term in (5.2) by $(1-p_n)^2$, we see that the adults in the $(n+1)$th generation are formed in the proportions

$$Su_n^2 AA : 2Su_n Aa : S(1-k)aa,$$

and hence
$$u_{n+1} = \frac{2Su_n^2 + 2Su_n}{2Su_n + 2S(1-k)} = \frac{u_n(u_n+1)}{u_n+1-k}. \qquad (5.3)$$

This is a recurrence relation which enables us to calculate the frequency of A genes in the $(n+1)$th generation in terms of the frequency in the nth generation. Knowing the initial frequency of gene A, and the 'selective disadvantage' k of aa, we could calculate the frequency of gene A in any subsequent generation by numerical iteration.

It would be convenient to find an analytical solution of (5.3), so that we could find for example u_{100} in terms of u_0 and k without the labour of 100 iterative steps. Unfortunately, this is not in general possible. However, it is possible to solve the important case when k

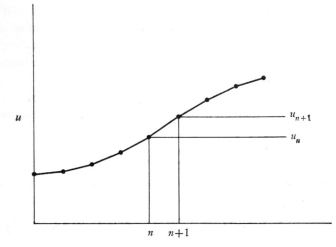

Fig. 21. The solution of a recurrence relation which could safely be replaced by a differential equation.

is small (say 0·01 or less). This we do by turning (5.3) into a differential equation—a procedure which is only justified when the change in u_n in one generation is not greatly different from the change in the preceding and in the following generation. Thus fig. 21 shows a possible graph of u_n against n which satisfies this condition. The graph consisting of a series of straight segments can safely be replaced by a continuously curving one whose slope at generation n is given by

$$\frac{u_{n+1}-u_n}{(n+1)-n} = u_{n+1}-u_n;$$

i.e. by a graph whose equation is

$$\frac{du_n}{dn} = u_{n+1} - u_n.$$

We will therefore replace equation (5.3) by

$$\frac{du_n}{dn} = u_{n+1} - u_n = \frac{ku_n}{u_n + 1 - k}. \tag{5.4}$$

Before attempting to solve (5.4), we note that if k is small, $u_{n+1} - u_n$ does not change rapidly with time, so it is safe to replace the recurrence relation by a differential equation. Also, if k is small, (5.4) can be replaced by

$$\frac{du_n}{dn} = \frac{ku_n}{u_n + 1}. \tag{5.5}$$

This is a differential equation with variables separate, so that

$$\int (1 + 1/u_n)\, du_n = k \int dn = kn.$$
$$\therefore \quad kn = [u_n + \ln u_n]_0^n$$
$$= u_n - u_0 + \ln \frac{u_n}{u_0}. \tag{5.6}$$

Thus suppose we have a recessive gene with a selective disadvantage of 1% ($k = 0.01$) and an initial frequency of 99.9%. Then $u_0 = \dfrac{0.001}{0.999} \simeq 0.001$, and hence

$$kn = u_n - 0.001 + \ln \frac{u_n}{0.001}. \tag{5.7}$$

From (5.7) we can calculate the number of generations taken for a given change in gene frequency, as shown in table 1.

Table 1

p_n	u_n	$\dfrac{u_n}{0.001}$	$\ln \dfrac{u_n}{0.001}$	kn	n
0.001	0.001	1	0	0	0
0.01	0.01	10	2.303	2.312	231
0.1	0.111	111	4.71	4.82	482
0.5	1.0	1,000	6.91	7.91	791
0.9	9	9,000	9.11	18.11	1811
0.99	99	99,000	11.52	110.52	11052
0.999	999	999,000	13.83	1012.83	101283

Thus with a 1 % advantage, an initially rare dominant gene will increase in frequency from 0·1 % to 10 % in 482 generations, from 10 to 90 % in 1329 generations, and will take almost one hundred thousand generations to increase from 90 to 99·9 %. The slowness with which the recessive is finally eliminated is due to the fact that a rare recessive is almost always present in heterozygotes, and so is not exposed to selection; for the same reason a rare but advantageous recessive gene increases in frequency very slowly.

c. Selection when all three genotypes have different fitnesses

If the fitnesses of the three genotypes have the relation

$$AA < Aa < aa,$$

then A will be replaced by a, as in the case when $AA = Aa < aa$, but at a greater rate, particularly when a is rare. But a novel type of behaviour arises when $AA < Aa > aa$; it will now be shown that an equilibrium exists with both A and a present in the population.

Let p be the frequency of gene A in the adult breeding population in the nth generation, and let $q = 1 - p$ be the frequency of a. Let the relative fitnesses of the three genotypes AA, Aa and aa be $1 - K : 1 : 1 - k$.

Then if N zygotes are formed by random mating, we have:

genotype	number of zygotes	number of surviving adults in generation $(n+1)$
AA	Np^2	$Np^2(1-K)$
Aa	$2Npq$	$2Npq$
aa	Nq^2	$Nq^2(1-k)$
Total	N	$N(1 - Kp^2 - kq^2)$.

Then the number of A genes in the adult population is

$$2Np^2(1-K) + 2Npq = 2Np(p - pK + q)$$

$$= 2Np(1 - pK).$$

Hence if p' is the frequency of gene A in the $n+1$th generation,

$$p' = \frac{2Np(1-pK)}{2N(1 - Kp^2 - kq^2)}. \tag{5.8}$$

Now if the population is in equilibrium, p does not change from generation to generation; i.e. $p = p'$, and so at equilibrium either

$$p = 0 \quad \text{or} \quad 1 - Kp^2 - kq^2 = 1 - pK.$$

Substituting $q = 1 - p$, and collecting terms in p^2 and p, this becomes

$$(K + k)p^2 - (K + 2k)p + k = 0,$$

$$\therefore \quad (p - 1)[(K + k)p - k] = 0,$$

or at equilibrium $\quad p = 0 \quad$ or $\quad 1 \quad$ or $\quad \dfrac{k}{K + k}.$ \hfill (5.9)

The equilibria at $p = 0$ and 1 are trivial, but that at $p = k/(K + k)$ is of great interest. An equilibrium is only meaningful if p lies between 0 and 1, and this requires that K and k have the same sign. Thus an equilibrium exists if the heterozygote is the fittest of the three genotypes, (K and k positive), or if the heterozygote is the least fit (K and k negative).

Are these equilibria stable? We can get a preliminary answer by asking how the gene frequency will change when A is rare, and when a is rare. Consider the case when K and k are positive. When A is rare, most A genes occur in heterozygotes (i.e. Aa is much commoner than AA). Then since k is positive, Aa is fitter than aa, and since AA is too rare to influence the result, A will increase in frequency. Similarly, when a is rare it will increase in frequency if K is positive.

It follows that when K and k are positive (i.e. the heterozygote is the fittest of the three genotypes) the equilibrium is stable; similarly, when K and k are negative, the equilibrium is unstable.

But this argument does not tell us whether, when K and k are positive, p will oscillate about its equilibrium value.

To settle this question we investigate small departures from the equilibrium.

In the nth generation, let $p = k/(K + k) + \delta$, where δ is a small departure from the equilibrium, and let $p' = k/(K + k) + \delta'$.

These values can be substituted in equation (5.8). After some algebraic manipulation, the resulting equation reduces to

$$\frac{k}{K + k} + \delta' = \left[\frac{k}{K + k} + \delta \right] \left[1 - K\delta \middle/ \left(1 - \frac{Kk}{K + k} \right) \right].$$

This can be further simplified if we remember that since δ is small, terms in δ^2 can be ignored. Hence

$$\delta' = \frac{K+k-2Kk}{K+k-Kk}\,\delta. \tag{5.10}$$

Let $\dfrac{K+k-2Kk}{K+k-Kk} = R$. Then if R lies between 0 and 1, the equilibrium is stable and non-oscillatory. In fact, when the heterozygote is the fittest of the three genotypes these conditions are satisfied. In this case, K and k are positive, but both must lie between 0 and 1, since if for example $K > 1$, then $1 - K$, the fitness of AA, would be negative, and negative fitnesses are meaningless. If K and k lie between 0 and 1, it is easy to verify that R also lies between 0 and 1.

If K and k are both negative, $R > 1$, and the equilibrium is unstable. If K and k have different signs, it has already been shown that no equilibrium exists.

D. The balance between selection and mutation

What will be the frequency of a gene which reduces fitness, but which is continuously reappearing by mutation?

This problem will first be solved for a deleterious dominant gene A, such that if the fitness of the 'normal' recessive homozygote aa is 1, the fitness of AA and Aa is $1 - K$. K is then a number between 0 and 1.

The 'mutation rate' from a to A will be taken as μ. This has the following meaning. Every gene present in a zygote has arisen by a series of replications from a gene present in the zygote from which one of its parents developed. The mutation rate μ is the probability that a mutation has taken place in this time interval of one generation.

Knowing μ and K, we want to find p_E, the equilibrium frequency of gene A. Before proceeding in detail, it will help to outline the method to be adopted:

(i) We assume that in one generation of zygotes the frequency of A is p and of a is q, where $p + q = 1$.

(ii) We then calculate successively the effects on p of selection and of mutation, and hence find the value p' of the frequency of A in the next generation of zygotes, in terms of μ and K.

(iii) We then argue that at equilibrium there is no change in gene frequency, and hence that $p = p' = p_E$.

In the initial population of zygotes, if mating is random, the genotype frequencies are $p^2 AA : 2pq\, Aa : q^2\, aa$. Thus if we start with a population of N zygotes and hence of $2N$ genes, we have after selection:

genotype	number after selection $\times 1/N$	gene	number after selection $\times 1/N$
AA	$p^2(1-K)$	A	$(2p^2+2pq)(1-K) = 2p(1-K)$
Aa	$2pq(1-K)$	a	$2q^2+2pq(1-K) = 2q - 2pqK$
aa	q^2	Total	$2 - 2Kp(1+q)$
Total	$1 - K(p^2+2pq)$		$= 2 - 2K(p^2+2pq)$

Note that the totals check; the number of genes is twice the number of individuals.

Mutation does not alter the total number of genes, but increases the number of A genes by $\mu(2q-2pqK)$, and decreases the number of a genes by the same amount. Hence after selection and mutation the frequency of A is

$$p' = \frac{2p(1-K)+2\mu q(1-pK)}{2-2K(p^2+2pq)}$$

$$= \frac{p - pK + \mu q - \mu pqK}{1 - Kp(p+2q)}. \qquad (5.11)$$

This expression can be greatly simplified if we make the assumption that p is very small. The assumption is justified because mutation rates are small (of the order of 10^{-5} or less) and hence genes which lower fitness can be maintained only at very low frequency by mutation.

If p is small, $1 - Kp(p+2q) \simeq 1$, and μpqK in the numerator is small compared to μq. Hence (5.11) becomes

$$p' = p - pK + \mu q,$$

and at equilibrium

$$p_E = p_E - Kp_E + \mu(1 - p_E),$$

or

$$p_E = \frac{\mu(1 - p_E)}{K} \simeq \frac{\mu}{K}. \qquad (5.12)$$

This simple result could have been reached more quickly if it had been assumed from the outset that p is small. Note that the assumption is justified provided that $\mu \ll K$.

Equation (5.12) sometimes enables us to determine mutation rates in human populations. Suppose we know F, the frequency at birth of an abnormality determined by a dominant gene A. Then provided that there is no difference in foetal mortality between normal and abnormal individuals, and that mating is random,

$$F = p^2 + 2pq \quad \text{or, if } p \text{ is small} \quad F \simeq 2p$$

and hence $$\mu = pK = \frac{FK}{2}. \tag{5.13}$$

Now if the fitness of affected individuals is very low—either through sterility or because they die before reaching reproductive age—then $K \simeq 1$, and the mutation rate μ equals half the frequency of abnormal births.

In the case of a rare and harmful recessive gene a, with frequency p, if the relative fitnesses of AA, Aa and aa are $1 : 1 : 1 - k$, it can be shown that at equilibrium $$\mu = kp^2. \tag{5.14}$$

If we again assume random mating and no foetal mortality, the frequency of abnormal births is p^2. However, we cannot use equation (5.14) to estimate mutation rates from known frequencies of abnormal births, for two reasons:

(i) Equation (5.14) assumes random mating. But in human populations cousin marriages, and other marriages between relatives, occur frequently enough to have a large effect on the frequency of individuals homozygous for rare genes (see p. 86, example 6). This could perhaps be allowed for, but:

(ii) It is impossible to be sure that AA and Aa have the same fitness. If Aa is only slightly fitter than AA, this would keep gene a at a frequency considerably higher than could be maintained by mutation alone.

E. Inbreeding

If two cousins marry, they may at any locus transmit to a child a pair of genes both of which are derived by successive replications from the same individual gene in one of the grandparents they have in common. In other words, two DNA molecules, each of which is a direct 'copy' of the same DNA molecule in an ancestor, may come together in a child.

In what follows, we will assume that two genes which are copies of the same gene in a recent ancestor are identical; that is, we will ignore the small probability that a mutation has occurred in the recent past. We will also assume that two genes at the same locus which are not copies of the same gene in a recent ancestor have a probability P_0 of being identical; in general, we do not know the value of P_0.

We will now define the 'coefficient of inbreeding' and the 'coefficient of parentage'.

I, the coefficient of inbreeding, is a property of an individual. It is the probability that, at any autosomal locus, the two genes present in that individual are identical.

R, the coefficient of parentage, is a property of two individuals. It is the probability that, at any autosomal locus, if one gene is drawn at random from each individual, those two genes will be identical. (For those already familiar with population genetics R corresponds to Malecot's *'coefficient de parente'* when $P_0 = 0$; I have used definitions of I and R which are unorthodox but which seem to me simpler to understand.)

It follows from these definitions that, if two individuals A and B have an offspring C, then

$$R_{AB} = I_C. \tag{5.15}$$

We will calculate first the value of I for individual C in the pedigree shown in fig. 22. C is in fact the offspring of a mating between half-sibs. Considering the two genes at any autosomal locus in C:

$$I_C = P_s + (1 - P_s)P_0,$$

where P_s is the probability that both genes in C are copies of the same gene in male G.

Consider the gene which C inherits from A: there is a probability of $\frac{1}{2}$ that this gene was inherited from G; if so, there is a probability of $\frac{1}{2}$ that G transmitted an identical gene to B; and if so, there is a probability of $\frac{1}{2}$ that B transmitted an identical gene to C.

Hence $\qquad\qquad P_s = (\tfrac{1}{2})^3,$

and $\qquad\qquad I_C = \tfrac{1}{8} + \tfrac{7}{8}P_0.$

The coefficient of parentage between half-sibs is likewise $\tfrac{1}{8} + \tfrac{7}{8}P_0$.

The argument whereby P_s was calculated can be generalised. It amounted to saying that a gene was certainly transmitted from A to C, and that for each of the steps $A-G$, $G-B$ and $B-C$, there

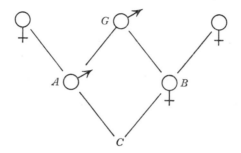

Fig. 22. Pedigree showing a mating between half sibs.

is a probability of $\tfrac{1}{2}$ that an identical gene was transmitted. The general proposition is then as follows:

If an individual C has parents A and B who have a common ancestor G, and if the 'loop' $C-A-X-Y-G-Z-B-C$ has n steps connecting parent and offspring, then

$$I_C = R_{AB} = (\tfrac{1}{2})^{n-1} + [1 - (\tfrac{1}{2})^{n-1}]P_0. \qquad (5.16)$$

What if there are two common ancestors, as in the pedigree in fig. 23, showing the mating of a bother and sister?

There are three mutually exclusive possibilities:

(i) the gene pair in C are copies of the same gene in G_1, with probability $(\tfrac{1}{2})^3 = \tfrac{1}{8}$;

(ii) the gene pair in C are copies of the same gene in G_2, with probability $\tfrac{1}{8}$;

(iii) the gene pair in C are not copies of a single gene in a recent ancestor, with probability $1 - \tfrac{1}{8} - \tfrac{1}{8} = \tfrac{3}{4}$.

Hence $\qquad I_C = R_{AB} = \tfrac{1}{8} + \tfrac{1}{8} + \tfrac{3}{4}P_0 = \tfrac{1}{4} + \tfrac{3}{4}P_0.$

We are now ready to tackle the problem of the rate of approach to homozygosity in a brother-sister mated line (fig. 24). Suppose that a male and female are selected from a large population to be the original parents (generation o) of such an inbred line, and that at N loci the 4 genes present (2 in each parent) are all different.

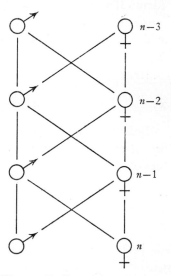

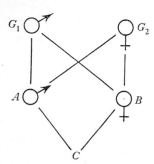

Fig. 23. Pedigree showing a mating between full sibs.

Fig. 24. Pedigree showing successive generations of brother-sister mating.

Then if for these loci I_n and R_n are the coefficients of inbreeding and parentage respectively in the nth generation, we have, remembering (5.15)

$$I_o = 0 \quad \text{and} \quad R_o = I_1 = 0. \qquad (5.17)$$

(If we supposed that the original parents were homozygous at all loci, but homozygous for different alleles at N loci, then for these loci our initial conditions would be $I_o = 1$ and $R_o = I_1 = 0$.)

We want to find I_n, the proportion of N originally segregating loci for which an individual in the nth generation is homozygous; since $I_n = R_{n-1}$, this will also give a measure of the genetic similarity between members of the population.

Consider a locus in an individual in the nth generation. There are three mutually exclusive possibilities:

(i) the two genes are copies of the same gene in the same grand-parent, with probability $\frac{1}{8}+\frac{1}{8}=\frac{1}{4}$; if so, the probability that they are identical is 1;

(ii) the two genes are copies of different genes in the same grandparent, with probability $\frac{1}{4}$; if so, the probability that they are identical is I_{n-2};

(iii) the two genes are copies of genes from different grandparents, with probability $\frac{1}{2}$; if so, the probability that they are identical is $R_{n-2}=I_{n-1}$.

Hence
$$I_n = \frac{1}{4}+\frac{1}{4}I_{n-2}+\frac{1}{2}I_{n-1},$$

or
$$4I_n = 1+I_{n-2}+2I_{n-1}. \tag{5.18}$$

Before finding an analytical solution of (5.18), its behaviour can be investigated numerically. Thus from (5.17) $I_0 = I_1 = 0$, and hence

$$I_2 = \tfrac{1}{4}(1+0+0) = 0.25$$

$$I_3 = \tfrac{1}{4}(1+0+0.5) = 0.375$$

$$I_4 = \tfrac{1}{4}(1+0.25+0.75) = 0.5$$

$$I_5 = \tfrac{1}{4}(1+0.375+1) = 0.594$$

$$I_6 = \tfrac{1}{4}(1+0.5+1.188) = 0.672 \quad \text{and so on.}$$

Thus after 6 generations of brother-sister mating, approximately two thirds of the initially segregating loci would be homozygous.

In seeking an analytical solution of (5.18), we notice that it closely resembles the equation solved in appendix 4, to which the solution had the form $x = A\lambda_1^n + B\lambda_2^n$. This will not quite do in the present case, because of the constant term. However, a solution of the form

$$I_n = 1 + A\lambda_1^n + B\lambda_2^n$$

will work, because when this is substituted in (5.18), the constant terms cancel out, and we are left with the requirement that λ_1 and λ_2 satisfy the equation
$$4\lambda^2 - 2\lambda - 1 = 0,$$

or
$$\lambda_1 = +0.808, \quad \lambda_2 = -0.308.$$

A and B can then be chosen to fit the initial conditions.

Thus if $\qquad I_0 = 0, \quad A + B = -1,$

and if $\qquad I_1 = 0, \quad 0.808A - 0.308B = -1,$

and hence $\qquad A = 1.172 \quad$ and $\quad B = 0.172.$

Hence $\qquad I_n = 1 - 1.172 \times 0.808^n + 0.172(-0.308)^n, \qquad$ (5.19)

and substituting various values of n:

generations	I_n
6	0.672 as before
10	0.861
50	$1 - 2.75 \times 10^{-5}$.

Examples

1 A *Drosophila* population cage is started by introducing 300 flies homozygous for the gene 'vestigial', 100 wild-type homozygotes, and 200 heterozygotes, each class consisting of equal number of males and females. Assuming random mating, write down the frequencies of different types of mating, and hence the proportions in which the three genotypes occur in the next generation. Check that these numbers agree with the Hardy–Weinberg ratio. What assumptions, other than random mating, have you made?

2 The ABO blood groups in man are determined by a system of 3 alleles, A, B and O. Genotypes AA and AO are group A, BB and BO are group B, AB is group AB, and OO is group O. The frequencies of the blood groups in England are 32.1 % A, 22.4 % B, 7.1 % AB and 38.4 % O. Are these proportions consistent with the assumption of random mating?

3 Homozygotes for a recessive gene r have a 2 % greater chance of survival than either R/R or R/r. The initial frequency of r in a random mating population is 1 per thousand. How many generations will elapse before the frequency of r reaches 50 %?

4 There is a gene S in man such that S/S individuals die soon after birth of anaemia. However, in areas where some $+/+$ individuals die of malaria as children, $S/+$ individuals never do. In an area of Africa, 10 % of adults are $S/+$. If this situation is stable, what proportion of $+/+$ individuals die of malaria in childhood? (The facts, concerning sickle-cell anaemia, have been simplified for the sake of the example.)

5 Derive equation (5.14).

6 What is the coefficient of parentage of first cousins? A harmful recessive gene is present in a population with a frequency of $1/200$. What is the frequency of homozygotes among the children of (a) unrelated parents, (b) first cousins?

7 An hermaphroditic organism reproduces by self-fertilisation. If an ancestral individual has a coefficient of inbreeding of I_0, what will be the coefficient of inbreeding n generations later?

6 TARGET THEORY

In several branches of biology, theories have been formulated which amount to saying that in each cell or in each organism there are a number of 'targets', and that changes occur as a consequence of random 'hits' on these targets. Such theories are most obviously relevant when explaining the effects of ionising radiations. By a natural extension, similar theories have been put forward to explain 'spontaneous' deteriorative changes, particularly those associated with senescence, and for the damaging effects of agents other than radiation.

This chapter introduces the mathematical methods used in developing these theories. There are two devices which are used again and again in target theory, but which have already been met in other contexts; they are as follows:

(1) If you can't calculate the probability that something will happen, calculate the probability that it won't.

(2) If x is small and n large, $(1-x)^n \simeq e^{-nx}$.

This identity, proved in appendix 6, was used on page 35 to analyse the 'random' meetings between a parasite and its host; it is used here to analyse the random collisions of ionising particles with their targets.

If these two devices are borne in mind, no great difficulty should be experienced in coping with the type of problem discussed in this chapter. As an inducement to those with no interest in radiation biology, the same mathematical ideas are used in many other contexts, particularly in ecology.

A. Single hit theories; mutagenesis

Suppose that a cell contains N targets, and that a hit on any one of these will kill the cell, or produce some other measurable effect. What proportion of cells will survive a given 'dose'—i.e. a given number of 'missiles' directed at it?

There are a number of biological problems to which the answer to this question might be relevant. Here are two of them:

(1) *Drosophila* sperm are bombarded with neutrons—the 'missiles'. The X chromosomes of these sperm contain a number of genes (the 'targets'), each of which is essential for normal development. There are breeding techniques which enable one to measure in what proportion of sperm one or more of these genes have mutated. How will this proportion vary with dose?

(2) An adult haploid insect (e.g. a male wasp) is treated with X-rays. Suppose that each cell contains N genes, each essential for its continued functioning. How will the proportion of cells rendered non-functional vary with dose?

In both these examples, the targets are genes. In a haploid cell there is only one copy of each gene, and hence a single hit is effective. There are a number of copies of most organelles—e.g. mitochondria, ribosomes—and hence single hits are unlikely to be effective. But there are other organs—e.g. the flagellum in some flagellates—of which there is only one per cell, and to which single hit models may be relevant.

Suppose that a cell containing N targets is exposed to a dose of K particles. Let the probability that a particular particle will hit a particular target be p; clearly p is very small.

The probability that a particular target is *not* hit by a particular particle is $1 - p$.

Hence the probability that a particular target is not hit by any of the K particles is:

$$(1 - p)^K \simeq e^{-Kp}.$$

Since there are N targets, if the probability that one target is hit is independent of the probability that any other target is hit, then the probability that no target is hit is $(e^{-Kp})^N = e^{-NKp}$.

There are two cases to be considered:

(1) The proportion of cells damaged is small. In this case NKp is small, and $e^{-NKp} \simeq 1 - NKp$. Hence the proportion of cells damaged is NKp; i.e. it is proportional to the dose. As an example, the proportion of sperm in which sex-linked lethal mutations are induced is (provided it is small) proportional to the dose of radiation.

(2) The proportion of cells undamaged is small. In this case the proportion of survivors, S, is e^{-NKp}.

Hence

$$\ln S = -NKp \qquad (6.1)$$

and the one hit theory implies that $\ln S$ should decline linearly with dose.

At this point, we have to consider more carefully what we mean by 'hits' on 'targets'.

Consider for example the effects of irradiating a virus or bacteriophage. Some 'hits'—i.e. alterations of the DNA—may be confined to a single 'functional unit' or cistron; if so, the viral DNA will no longer be able to code for one particular protein, but its ability to code for all other proteins will be unaltered. If this is the type of hit which is relevant, then the number of targets in a virus equals the number of cistrons—i.e. the number of regions of DNA specifying distinct proteins. However, other alterations may make it impossible for the viral DNA to be replicated. In this case, each virus is a single target.

It follows that in any particular experimental situation, there may be different numbers of targets of different 'sizes' and probabilities of being hit. Provided that a single hit on any target will kill the organism, then it remains true that $\ln S$ declines linearly with dose.

Thus suppose a dose of K particles is used, and that there are n_1 targets such that the probability that a particular particle hits a particular target is p_1, and n_2 targets such that the probability that a particular particle hits a particular target is p_2. Then the probability that no target is hit is given by:

$$S = e^{-n_1 K p_1} \cdot e^{-n_2 K p_2} \quad \text{or} \quad \ln S = -(n_1 p_1 + n_2 p_2) K,$$

and as before, $\ln S$ declines linearly with dose.

B. Multi-hit theories

Suppose now that in each cell there are r targets of each of N different kinds. If $r = 3$, this could be represented as follows:

$$A\ B\ C\text{.....................}N,$$
$$A\ B\ C\text{.....................}N,$$
$$A\ B\ C\text{.....................}N.$$

Suppose also that the cell dies if all r targets of any one kind are hit. Examples are as follows:

(1) A triploid cell ($r = 3$) contains N gene loci essential for its continued survival. Damage to genes is recessive; i.e. so long as one undamaged gene remains at each locus, the cell survives.

(2) A bacterium is infected by r similar bacteriophages, each containing N essential genes. Provided that at each of the N loci one gene is undamaged, a functional bacteriophage can be produced by recombination. What dose of radiation will prevent this?

As before, the probability that any one target is hit after a dose K is $1 - e^{-pK}$.

Hence, assuming independence, the probability that at any locus all r targets are hit is $(1 - e^{-pK})^r$.

Hence at any locus the probability that at least one gene remains undamaged is:
$$1 - (1 - e^{-pK})^r.$$

Hence the probability that at least one gene remains undamaged at all N loci is:
$$S = [1 - (1 - e^{-pK})^r]^N$$

where S is the proportion of surviving cells. Provided that the probability that any particular target escapes is small, i.e. that e^{-pK} is small:
$$S = (1 - 1 + r e^{-pK})^N = r^N e^{-NpK}.$$

Therefore
$$\ln S = N \ln r - NpK. \tag{6.2}$$

Equation (6.2) has been used in the study of viral replication within a bacterium. Thus suppose that a bacterium is infected by a single virus particle. The viral *DNA* is replicated, so that after say x minutes there are r copies of the virus within the bacterium. The bacterium is then treated with ultraviolet light. If the dose is sufficient to knock out all r particles, then the bacterium is no longer 'infective'—i.e. it will no longer infect other bacteria with the virus.

Thus in this experiment S is the fraction of bacteria which are infective. Since we have assumed that a single hit destroys a viral particle, $N = 1$, and from (6.2) $\ln S = \ln r - pK$. Therefore if our theory is correct we would expect $\ln S$ to vary with dose and with time after infection as shown in fig. 25. Ideally, we should be able to tell from such an experiment how many copies of the original virus have been made a given number of minutes after infection.

Fig. 26 *a* shows the results of such an experiment on bacteriophage T7 in the bacterium *E. coli*. They agree rather well with theory. The curves at different times after infection have the same slope at high dosages, but the later curves have a 'shoulder' indicating a multi-

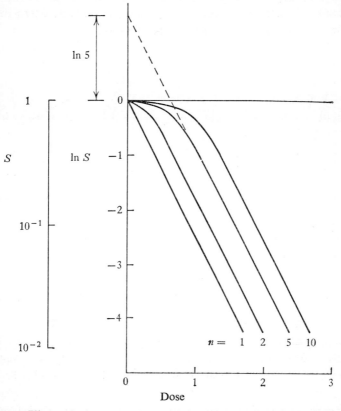

Fig. 25. Theoretical curves of infectivity (*S*) as a function of dose, for varying numbers *n* = 1, 2, 5 and 10 of bacteriophage particles per bacterium.

plicity of targets. The agreement is not exact: the 7-minute curve, for example, has the shape to be expected if different bacteria contain different numbers of phage particles.

Fig. 26 *b* shows the results of a similar experiment on bacteriophage T2. It does not agree at all with the predictions of the theory.

A likely explanation for this discrepancy is as follows: phage T2 can undergo genetic recombination within the bacterium. Suppose therefore there are 4 phage particles in a bacterium, and all have been hit. Provided that they have not been hit in the same place, there is a possibility that genetic recombination may give rise to an undamaged particle. Consequently infectivity remains after a much higher dose than would otherwise be the case.

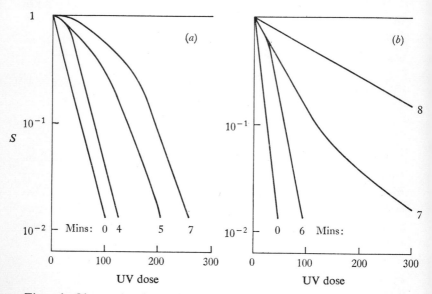

Fig. 26. Observed values of infectivity (S) against dose, for bacteria irradiated varying numbers of minutes after infection. (a) bacteriophage T7; (b) bacteriophage T2. (After Benzer, S. (1952). *J. Bact.* **63**, 59.)

It is characteristic of mathematical ideas in biology that they are most suggestive when they are contradicted by experiment. In the present case, the difference between fig. 26a and b suggests the possibility of viral recombination; in the absence of a mathematical theory, there would be no reason to regard fig. 26b as in any way anomalous.

In the above example, we calculated the probability that each of r identical targets would receive one hit. In other cases we want to know the probability that a particular target will be hit r times. For example, the origin of an inversion requires that a chromosome be hit and broken at least twice. This is because broken ends of chromosomes tend to join up again, so that after two breaks the middle piece may be inverted relative to the ends.

Suppose that the probability that a particular chromosone is broken by a particular particle is p, where p is small. Then the probability that the chromosome is not broken by a dose k is $(1-p)^k$.

We will consider only the case in which the dose k is such that in most cells no chromosomes are broken; i.e. that $(1-p)^k \simeq 1$.

By the binomial theorem (p. 61) the probability that the chromosome is broken exactly twice is

$$\frac{k(k-1)}{2}p^2(1-p)^{k-2} \simeq \frac{k^2p^2}{2}(1-p)^k$$

$$\simeq \tfrac{1}{2}k^2p^2. \tag{6.3}$$

And since the number of cells with more than two breaks will be small compared to the number with exactly two, the frequency of inversions will be proportional to the square of the dose k. This conclusion holds only if the frequency is small; it should be compared with our earlier conclusion that the frequency of sex-linked recessive mutations would be proportional to the dose.

c. The Poisson series

This example leads to a modification of the binomial theorem which is of common application in biology. The binomial theorem states that if the probability of a success in a single trial is p, then the probabilities of 0, 1, 2, 3, ... successes out of n trials are given by successive terms in the series:

$$q^n + npq^{n-1} + \frac{n(n-1)}{2}p^2q^{n-2} + \frac{n(n-1)(n-2)}{3!}p^3q^{n-3} + \dots$$

$$= q^n \left[1 + n\frac{p}{q} + \frac{n(n-1)}{2}\left(\frac{p}{q}\right)^2 + \frac{n(n-1)(n-2)}{3!}\left(\frac{p}{q}\right)^3 + \dots \right].$$

$$\tag{6.4}$$

Now suppose that p is very small, but n is large so that np is not negligible. Then (6.4) can be replaced by

$$(1-p)^n \left(1 + np + \tfrac{1}{2}(np)^2 + \frac{1}{3!}(np)^3 + \ldots\right)$$

$$= e^{-np} \left(1 + np + \tfrac{1}{2}(np)^2 + \frac{1}{3!}(np)^3 + \ldots\right). \quad (6.5)$$

Notice that the expression inside the bracket is e^{np}, and hence the sum of all the terms in (6.5) is unity; the terms represent the probabilities that there are 0, 1, 2, 3, ... successes out of n trials, and their sum is necessarily unity.

Series (6.5) is known as the Poisson series. It is important in many branches of biology. It can be applied wherever it is possible to imagine that a large number n independent trials have been made, the probability of a success in any trial being small. Clearly the average number of successes m out of n trials is given by $m = np$. The Poisson series states that the probabilities of 0, 1, 2, ..., r, ... successes out of n trials are:

Number of successes	0	1	2	...	r	...
probability	e^{-m}	$m\,e^{-m}$	$\tfrac{1}{2}m^2 e^{-m}$	...	$\frac{1}{r!}m^r e^{-m}$	....

It has already been shown that the sum of these probabilities is unity. We will now satisfy ourselves that the average number of successes is, as stated above, equal to m.

The average number of successes is

$$0 \times e^{-m} + 1 \times m\,e^{-m} + 2 \times \tfrac{1}{2}m^2 e^{-m} + \ldots + \frac{r}{r!}m^r e^{-m} + \ldots$$

$$= m\,e^{-m}\left(1 + m + \ldots + \frac{1}{(r-1)!}m^{r-1} + \ldots\right)$$

$$= m \quad \text{as required.}$$

When studying radiation, it is natural to think of missiles hitting targets. The same mathematics can be applied to problems where the missile–target analogy is less obviously appropriate. Suppose for example that a large population of N bacteria is mixed with a population of kN phage particles. If it is assumed that all phage particles enter a bacterium, infection being random, what proportion of bacteria escape infection? The inverse of this problem may also arise: if a fraction F of the bacteria escape infection, what is k, the average number of phage particles per bacterium?

We regard the bacteria as targets, and the phage particles as missiles. Then the probability that a particular bacterium will be infected by a particular phage is $1/N$. Hence the probability that the bacterium will escape infection altogether is $(1-1/N)^{kN} = e^{-k}$. Further, the proportion of bacteria infected by 0, 1, 2, ... phage particles are

$$e^{-k}(1 + k + k^2/2 + k^3/3! + \ldots).$$

A similar application arises when counting cells on a grid. Suppose, for example, that blood containing N red cells is spread on a glass slide, whose surface is divided by a square grid into 400 equal areas. Provided that the cells are distributed randomly over the slide, the probability that a particular cell falls into a particular square is $1/400$, and hence the expected numbers of squares with 0, 1, 2, ... cells are

$$400\,e^{-N/400}\left[1 + \frac{N}{400} + \frac{1}{2}\left(\frac{N}{400}\right)^2 + \frac{1}{3!}\left(\frac{N}{400}\right)^3 + \ldots\right].$$

If, for example, 61 of the 400 cells contained no red cells, then

$$400\,e^{-N/400} \simeq 61 \quad \text{or} \quad N \simeq 752.$$

Provided that it is known that the cells are randomly distributed, this affords a quick way of estimating their number.

D. Ecological applications

In ecology, the Poisson series is used to discover whether organisms are in fact randomly distributed in space. A given area is divided by a grid into a large number of small squares, and the numbers of individuals of a particular animal or plant species in each square are counted. Alternatively, if the region is too large to be treated in this way, a number of squares are chosen at random, and the numbers of individuals in them are counted. In either case, the numbers of squares containing 0, 1, 2, ... individuals are compared with the numbers expected according to the Poisson series. If the observed and expected numbers agree reasonably well, it is concluded that the distribution is near enough random. The alternatives to a random distribution are:

(1) Individuals avoid one another, or prevent the establishment of other individuals close to them. In such cases, if for example the average number per square were three, there would be too many squares with exactly three individuals and too few either with no individuals or with a large number.

(2) Individuals are clumped together—perhaps because they attract one another, or because only some parts of the region provide suitable conditions for them. In such cases there will be too many empty squares and too many squares with large numbers.

The logic behind this argument is that if the cells on a glass slide or the thistles in a field are randomly distributed, then their distribution is similar to that obtained by the following process:

(i) Divide the region up into a large number of small squares of equal area.

(ii) Place the individuals one by one into squares by a random process (e.g. number off the squares and choose the numbers by spinning a roulette wheel). In doing this, the probability of choosing a square should be the same for all squares, and should be unaffected by whether the square already contains one or more individuals.

Examples

1 543 bottles were collected in the neighbourhood of a lay-by. In some of these were found the remains of small mammals which had entered the bottle and been unable to get out again. The numbers were:

Number of mammals in each bottle	0	1	2	3	4	5	6	7
Number of bottles	468	41	16	11	2	4	0	1

Are some bottles more likely to trap small mammals than others? If not, and if the same total number of mammals had been trapped, how many empty bottles would you expect there to be?

2 A lawn is divided into 900 equal squares. 221 of these squares contain no daisies. If daisies are randomly distributed over the lawn, how many squares would you expect to contain 3 daisies?

3 According to a particular theory of ageing, recessive mutations occur in the nuclei of non-dividing cells. A cell dies *either* when both alleles at any locus have mutated, *or*, in individuals initially heterozygous for a recessive lethal at any locus, when the other allele at that locus mutates. When a fraction f of the cells initially present have died, the individual dies.

If for all loci the probability that a mutation will occur in a short time is $\mu \Delta t$, prove that the probability that a gene will have mutated at age t is $1 - e^{-\mu t}$, which equals μt if μt is small.

In a particular species, 500 loci, all diploid, are essential for the continued life of the cell. The life span of individuals carrying no recessive lethals is L_0. Prove that

$$L_0 \simeq \frac{1}{\mu} \sqrt{\frac{-\ln(1-f)}{500}}.$$

If L_n is the life span of individuals initially heterozygous for n recessive lethals, show that

$$n\mu L_n + (500-n)\,\mu^2 L_n^2 = -\ln(1-f).$$

If $L_n = \frac{1}{2}L_0$ and $f = 0 \cdot 1$, find n.

4 A particular disease is incurable but does not alter the expectation of life. According to one theory, it develops if dominant mutations have occurred at two different loci in any one of a large number of 'immunologically competent' cells. If the mutation rates and the cell number are constant with age, how will the 'prevalence' P (i.e. the proportion of people affected) vary with age t?

A. The control of muscular movement

To illustrate the problem of control, we will consider the control of
limb movements. How is it, for example, that I am able to lift a spoon
and put it in my mouth?

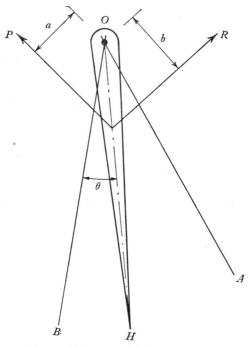

Fig. 27. Diagram of limb movement.

The problem is shown diagrammatically in fig. 27.

A limb OH rotates about point O; in practice there may be several
joints (e.g. shoulder, elbow and wrist), but this complicates the
problem without altering it in principle. The limb is being moved

from an initial position OA to a 'goal' position OB; it is convenient to measure its position by the angle θ between the actual and goal positions. It is moved by a muscle exerting a force P at a distance a from the pivot O, and the movement is opposed by an antagonistic muscle exerting a force R at a distance b from O.

Hence the couple accelerating the limb in a clockwise direction (θ decreasing) is $Pa - Rb$, and hence if I is the moment of inertia of the limb about the pivot O,

$$Pa - Rb = -I\frac{d^2\theta}{dt^2}$$

or

$$I\frac{d^2\theta}{dt^2} + Pa - Rb = 0. \qquad (7.1)$$

a and b will alter slightly as the limb rotates, but the nature of the problem is unaffected by these alterations, and we will assume that a and b are constants and equal to one another.

Clearly, if the limb is to finish in position OB, P and R must vary with θ, and when $\theta = 0$, $Pa - Rb = a(P - R) = 0$. Now P and R depend immediately on the nature of the messages travelling down the motor nerves supplying the muscles. In some way therefore these messages must be made to depend on θ, and hence information must be supplied to the brain or spinal cord about θ. For the moment, we will accept that such information exists without enquiring about its nature.

The simplest assumptions we can make which satisfy the condition $Pa - Rb = 0$ when $\theta = 0$ is that $R = 0$ and $P = k\theta$ when θ is positive, and that $P = 0$ and $R = -k\theta$ when θ is negative; i.e. we assume that if a muscle is extended from the length it would have in the goal position, it exerts a force proportional to its extension. Equation (7.1) then becomes

$$\frac{d^2\theta}{dt^2} + \frac{ka}{I}\theta = 0 \qquad (7.2)$$

which has a solution (see appendix 5) of the form

$$\theta = A\sin\sqrt{\frac{ks}{I}}\, t \qquad (7.3)$$

i.e. an undamped oscillation.

Clearly, we must allow for a more complicated relation between P and R, and θ. The muscle which at any moment is not being stimulated to contract will nevertheless present some resistance to motion owing to its viscosity. This viscous resistance would result in a gradual damping of the oscillation described by (7.3), but is too small to explain the highly damped movements which limbs can make. It will be ignored here for simplicity.

Since the simplest assumption leads to an undamped oscillation, we have to make more complex assumptions about the way P and R depend on θ. For the moment we will make the quite general assumption that

$$P = f_1(\theta); \quad R = f_2(\theta). \tag{7.4}$$

Then $Pa - Rb = af_1(\theta) - bf_2(\theta) = F(\theta)$ say. In other words, the couple moving the limb depends on θ. We also know that when $\theta = 0$, $F(\theta) = 0$. We can now use a trick we have used several times before; for small displacements we can replace the actual function $F(\theta)$ by a straight line; for small displacements, $F(\theta) = C\theta$, where C is a constant, and hence equation (7.1) becomes

$$I\frac{d^2\theta}{dt^2} + C\theta = 0. \tag{7.5}$$

In other words, the limb will still oscillate either side of the goal position. Thus even though we have allowed for the force in the antagonistic muscles, and have permitted the forces P and R in the main and antagonistic muscles to vary with θ in any way whatever, we still reach the conclusion that the limb will oscillate either side of its target, although our conclusion now only holds for small displacements.

How then can a limb be designed which will approach its goal position without oscillations? Or to be pedantic, what features will have been incorporated by natural selection because they prevent oscillations? Any engineer will at once know the answer to this question. We must incorporate into the system a force which varies, not with the displacement θ, but with the velocity of movement, $d\theta/dt$.

Still without bothering about how this is to be achieved, we will assume that the two muscles are able to produce a couple with two components, one of which acts so as to move the limb towards its goal position and is proportional to the displacement θ, and the other of which acts so as to oppose the movement of the limb and is proportional to the velocity $d\theta/dt$. Hence the couple acting in a clockwise direction is

$$k\theta + l\frac{d\theta}{dt},$$

and hence

$$I\frac{d^2\theta}{dt^2} + l\frac{d\theta}{dt} + k\theta = 0, \qquad (7.6)$$

where k and l are positive constants.

The solution of this equation (see appendix 5) is

$$\theta = \exp\left(-\frac{l}{2I}t\right)\left\{A\exp\left(\frac{\sqrt{[l^2-4kI]}}{2I}t\right) + B\exp\left(-\frac{\sqrt{[l^2-4kI]}}{2I}t\right)\right\}$$

$$(7.7)$$

where A and B are constants.

Clearly l must be positive if the limb is to come to rest.

If $l^2 > 4kI$, θ will decrease without change of sign; i.e. the movement of the limb is non-oscillatory.

If $l^2 < 4kI$, then it is shown in appendix 5 that (7.7) can be written in the form

$$\theta = \exp\left(-\frac{l}{2I}t\right)\left\{\alpha\cos\frac{\sqrt{[4kI-l^2]}}{2I}t + \beta\sin\frac{\sqrt{[4kI-l^2]}}{2I}t\right\} \quad (7.8)$$

where α and β are constants. (7.8) describes an oscillation of decreasing amplitude.

Thus to eliminate oscillations requires $l^2 \geqslant 4kI$, when $l\,d\theta/dt$ is the force decelerating the limb, $k\theta$ the force moving it towards its goal, and I its moment of inertia.

So far we have assumed that P and R can be made to depend on θ and $d\theta/dt$ without enquiring how this is to be brought about, except that it was made clear that it requires sensory input, because the viscous resistance to motion is too small to be effective in damping. There are in fact four kinds of sensory information which could be relevant:

(i) We can see where our limbs are. But since I can put a spoon in my mouth in the dark, visual information cannot be necessary.

(ii) There are sense organs in the tendons, which measure the forces P and R directly. The sense endings have a high threshold, and probably are not involved in the accurate control of movement; they may be important in preventing a limb being over-stressed.

(iii) There are sense organs in the joints, which measure the displacement θ directly. They do not acclimatise quickly, and may therefore be important mainly in enabling a limb to be held in a fixed position.

(iv) There are sense organs in the muscles themselves. These 'muscle spindles' are shown diagrammatically in fig. 28.

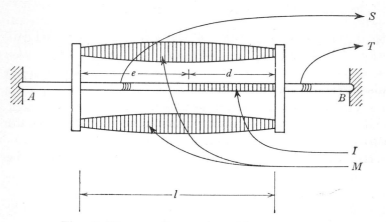

Fig. 28. Diagram of a muscle and its sense organs.

In this figure, the muscle is attached to its origin and insertion, A and B, by tendons. Two muscle fibres are shown, and between them the muscle spindle. The latter consists of two parts in series, a contractile part of length d and a sensory part of length e, so that $d+e = l$, the length of a muscle fibre. Two kinds of efferent nerve fibre carry messages to the muscle: M is the motor nerve causing the muscle to contract, and I the 'intrafusal' nerve fibre causing the contractile part of the spindle to contract. There are two kinds of afferent nerve fibres: T providing information about the tension in the tendon, and S providing information about changes in the length e.

Consider first what happens when a limb is held stationary by a balance between antagonistic muscles. If the limb moves so as to stretch a muscle, then l and e increase. Any increase in e causes an increase in the frequency of impulses in nerve S, and by a spinal reflex this causes nerve M to stimulate the muscle to contract. The 'knee jerk' reflex is mediated in this way; a blow to the tendon stretches the muscle spindle, and the muscle contracts in response.

One way in which a controlled movement of the limb could be produced is as follows. Suppose that the movement requires that the length l be reduced by an amount Δl. Then the first event could be a message travelling down nerve I causing a reduction in length d by Δl; there is evidence that sometimes the first event in the movement of a limb is such a message. This may seem to be merely transferring the difficulty; if a message in I can cause d to shorten by Δl, why not a message in M causing l to alter by Δl directly? The reason is simple; virtually no inertia is associated with changes in d, but there is considerable viscous damping, and so messages in I will not lead to oscillations. If d is decreased by Δl, then e is increased by Δl, and messages announcing this fact will travel along S. Messages will then be sent along M until e has been restored to its original value by reducing l.

It has already been shown that messages in M must depend not only on e, but also on de/dt, if the movement is to be non-oscillatory. There are two ways in which this could be done:

(i) the frequency of impulses in S may depend solely on e, increasing as e increases. The central nervous system could then perform a process of 'differentiation', responding not only to the frequency of impulses in S, but also to the rate of change of that frequency;

(ii) the muscle spindle itself may be such that the distortion of the relevant part of it, and hence the message in S, depends not only on e but also on de/dt.

In fact both these mechanisms probably operate.

To summarise, controlled and non-oscillatory movements are possible because the forces P and R are adjusted so that they depend both on θ and $d\theta/dt$, this adjustment depending on information about θ received from the muscle spindles.

It is instructive to compare this method of preventing 'overshooting' and oscillation with that which would be adopted by an engineer, at least by an old-fashioned engineer. The engineer would also generate a force R which was a function of the velocity of movement, but he would probably do so by inserting some kind of viscous damping device—for example a piston which can only move into a cylinder by forcing oil through a narrow space. For example, if an aeroplane lands heavily it is prevented from bouncing off again by the presence of such a device in its undercarriage. If all we wanted to do with our arms was to push food into our mouths, then a viscous damping device might be quite satisfactory. But sometimes we want to produce a very rapid movement, without being too worried by the possibility of an overshoot. For example, we may wish to strike an enemy on the jaw. In any such action a viscous damping device would be a grave disadvantage. But if the term $b\,d\theta/dt$ depends on sensory input along S, then in an emergency this input can be ignored, and messages can be sent along M causing maximum muscle contraction regardless of the messages in S.

However, a skilful boxer would not risk everything on a single blow. If he misses he does not wish to fall over, and in fact his fist will stop only a few inches beyond the point at which he had hoped to connect with his opponent's jaw. How is this to be achieved, if information in S is, at least initially, being ignored?

A possible answer is as follows. With experience, one can learn that a particular sequence of messages sent along the motor nerves supplying both the main and antagonistic muscles will produce a particular result. Clearly one would have to learn not only the sequence in which the messages were to be sent, but also the exact time intervals between them. Most training in athletic and other muscular skills probably has as its function the impressing on the central nervous system of a number of such 'programmes', known by experience to produce particular movements.

In the case of limb movements, the main factor tending to cause overshooting and oscillation is inertia; i.e. the fact that a limb once moving will continue to move until something stops it. Delays in the feedback loop play a lesser, though sometimes significant role. There is no analogue of inertia in most biological systems: a population which has been increasing has no inherent tendency to continue to do so if conditions change, except in so far as its age structure may cause a delay in its response. Similarly, a gene which has been increasing in frequency will start to decrease immediately if it is selected against. In the same way, there is no 'inertia' associated with chemical reactions, whose rates can change instantaneously if conditions are changed. The clearest analogue of inertia is the inductance of a coil in electromagnetism; if a current is flowing in a coil, it produces a magnetic field which tends to oppose any reduction in the current. It is for this reason that it is easy to build an oscillating electrical circuit, and that the behaviour of mechanical systems can be deduced from the behaviour of analogous electrical circuits.

B. The kinetics of chemical reactions

A feedback system similar to that concerned with the control of muscular movements is illustrated by the control of protein synthesis. But before we can write down the appropriate equations, we must have some idea of how the rates of chemical reactions vary with the concentrations of the reacting substances.

Consider first a reaction in which a compound breaks up into two components; i.e. $AB \rightarrow A + B$. If a single AB molecule is to break up, it must be supplied with a sufficiently large packet of energy, the so-called 'activation energy'. At a constant temperature, the probability that a particular AB molecule will receive a large enough packet of energy in a given time is constant. Hence the rate of the reaction $AB \rightarrow A + B$ is simply proportional to the number of AB molecules, i.e. to the concentration of AB.

Now consider the reverse reaction, $A + B \rightarrow AB$. Again a certain minimum energy (not necessarily the same) is required to initiate the reaction. The situation as far as energy is concerned is shown in fig. 29, for a case in which heat is liberated when A and B combine to form AB.

For a particular A molecule, the probability that it will combine with a B molecule in a given time is equal to the probability that it will collide with a B molecule, multiplied by the probability that a given collision will be associated with an energy greater than the activation energy. At a constant temperature, the latter probability is constant, and the probability of a collision is proportional to the concentration of B molecules. Thus at a constant temperature the rate of the reaction $A + B \rightarrow AB$ is proportional to the product of the concentrations of A and B.

To see how rates of reaction vary with temperature, we need to know how the energies of molecules are distributed. Not all molecules are in the same state; some are moving faster than others, and some are vibrating more energetically. According to Boltzmann's principle (the derivation is beyond the scope of this book), if N molecules are present in a system in equilibrium, and of these N_E have an energy greater than or equal to E, then

$$N_E/N = e^{-E/RT}, \tag{7.9}$$

where R is the gas constant and T the absolute temperature.

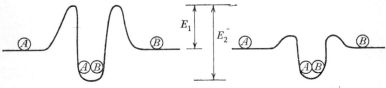

With enzyme

Fig. 29. Energy contours for the reaction $A + B \rightleftharpoons AB$, with and without enzyme catalysis.

Consider now the reversible reaction $A + B \rightleftharpoons AB$, where x_A, x_B and x_{AB} are the relevant concentrations, and E_1 and E_2 are the activation energies of the reactions $A + B \rightarrow AB$ and $AB \rightarrow A + B$ respectively. The reaction $A + B \rightarrow AB$ then releases a quantity of heat $E_2 - E_1$. The frequency of collisions between A and B molecules is $Cx_A x_B$, where C will depend on the velocities with which the molecules are moving. It can be shown that over the range of temperatures characteristic of biological systems the velocities do not change very much, and so C can be taken as a constant. The proportion of collisions associated with an energy greater than E_1 is $e^{-E_1/RT}$, and hence the rate of the reaction $A + B \rightarrow AB$ is

$$Cx_A x_B e^{-E_1/RT}. \tag{7.10}$$

By a similar argument, the proportion of AB molecules associated with an energy greater than E_2 is $e^{-E_2/RT}$, and hence the rate of the reaction $AB \rightarrow A + B$ is

$$C'x_{AB}e^{-E_2/RT}. \tag{7.11}$$

At equilibrium, the two rates are equal, and hence

$$\frac{x_A x_B}{x_{AB}} = K e^{(E_1 - E_2)/RT}, \tag{7.12}$$

where $K = C'/C$ does not vary greatly with temperature.

Note that the equilibrium depends on temperature. At a constant temperature, $x_A x_B / x_{AB}$ is constant. It follows that the proportion of substance A which is not combined—i.e. $x_A/(x_A + x_{AB})$—is not a constant, but increases as the substances are diluted.

(7.10), (7.11) and (7.12) describe the reaction in the absence of an enzyme. An enzyme acts by reducing the activation energies E_1 and E_2; i.e. by reducing the height of the 'rim' round the 'hole' in fig. 29. By reducing the activation energy, an enzyme increases the proportion of collisions which are associated with an adequate energy, and so increases the rate of reaction.

However, an enzyme cannot alter the energy released by a reaction, $E_2 - E_1$; if it could, then enzymes could be used to construct a perpetual motion machine. It follows from (7.12) that an enzyme does not alter the equilibrium value of $x_A x_B / x_{AB}$.

Finally, we can ask how the rates of reaction will vary with temperature. We will compare the rates k_1 and k_2 of the reaction $A + B \rightarrow AB$ at the two temperatures T_1 and T_2. Then

$$k_2/k_1 = Cx_A x_B e^{-E_1/RT_2} \div Cx_A x_B e^{-E_1/RT_1}$$

$$= \exp\left[\frac{E_1}{R}\left(\frac{1}{T_1} - \frac{1}{T_2}\right)\right]. \tag{7.13}$$

From which it follows that the greater the activation energy E_1, the greater will be the change in the rate of reaction for a given change of temperature.

c. The control of protein synthesis

The simplest possible model for the control of protein synthesis is shown in fig. 30.

In this figure, messenger RNA is made in the nucleus. Its concentration at any moment is Y. At the ribosomes the 'message' is translated, and enzyme molecules synthesised; their concentration is Z. This enzyme then catalyses the reaction from an inactive precursor, concentration P, to a repressor molecule, concentration M. The repressor molecule then reacts with the gene, so that when a repressor is attached to a gene no mRNA is made.

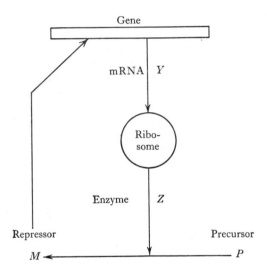

Fig. 30. A simple mechanism for regulating gene action.

This is the simplest form of such a control system. How will it behave? To answer this question, we need to know how Y, Z and M change with time; i.e. we need expressions for dY/dt, dZ/dt and dM/dt.

(i) An equation for dY/dt.

The number of genes in a cell is constant (2 in a diploid). Hence the rate of synthesis of Y will depend on the proportion of time, p, for which the gene is uncombined with repressor. This proportion p is the same as the proportion of genes, in a large population N (i.e. in $N/2$ cells), which at any instant are not combined with repressor. Then the number of genes with repressor attached is $N(1-p)$, and there is a constant probability a that any particular repressor molecule will become detached in a given time interval. Hence the rate at which repressor molecules are being detached is $aN(1-p)$.

The number of unrepressed genes is Np. Hence the rate at which repressor molecules are attaching to unrepressed genes is proportional to the product of their concentrations; i.e. to MNp.

Hence at equilibrium

$$aN(1-p) = bMNp,$$

or the fraction of unrepressed genes is

$$p = a/(a+bM).$$

Whence the rate of synthesis of mRNA is $c/(a+bM)$, where a, b and c are constants:

The rate at which mRNA molecules are lost or destroyed is likely to be proportional to their concentration. If so

$$\frac{dY}{dt} = \frac{c}{a+bM} - kY. \qquad (7.14)$$

(ii) An equation for dZ/dt.

Provided there is an adequate supply of ribosomes, the rate of synthesis of enzyme will be proportional to the concentration of the corresponding mRNA. Also, the rate of loss of enzyme will be proportional to its own concentration. Hence

$$\frac{dZ}{dt} = eY - fZ, \qquad (7.15)$$

where e and f are constants.

(iii) An equation for dM/dt.

We will write Pr, Enz and Rp for the precursor, enzyme and repressor respectively. If the reaction catalysed by the enzyme is $Pr \rightarrow Rp + A$, where A is some other reaction product, then the first step is for the enzyme to combine with the precursor, and the second for this compound to break up into enzyme, repressor and reactant A. The full sequence is then

$$Enz + Pr \rightarrow (Enz\text{-}Pr) \rightarrow Enz + Rp + A.$$

In this sequence, the first step usually proceeds much more

rapidly than the second, which is therefore rate-limiting. Hence provided that Pr is present in adequate concentration, most enzyme molecules will be bound to precursor, and hence the rate of production of repressor will be proportional to the concentration of the enzyme.

Hence if, as is reasonable, the rate of removal of repressor is proportional to its concentration,

$$\frac{dM}{dt} = gZ - hM, \tag{7.16}$$

where g and h are constants.

At this stage we have three equations, and three unknowns, Y, Z and M. However, we can simplify things a little by the following considerations. The reaction $Pr \rightarrow Rp$ is a single enzyme-catalysed step, whereas the synthesis of both mRNA and protein involves a long and complex sequence of reactions. Therefore equation (7.16) will reach its equilibrium point much more rapidly than (7.14) and (7.15). Hence if we are interested in changes in Y and Z, we can safely assume that M has at any instant its equilibrium value for the contemporary values of Y and Z. Thus in (7.16) we assume that $dM/dt = 0$, and hence that $M = gZ/h$.

Substituting in (7.14), and writing $bg/h = l$, we obtain

$$\left. \begin{aligned} \frac{dY}{dt} &= \frac{c}{a+lZ} - kY, \\ \frac{dZ}{dt} &= eY - fZ. \end{aligned} \right\} \tag{7.17}$$

The important question about these equations is whether they give rise to a sustained oscillation, or whether any disturbance is rapidly damped out.

To answer this question, we go through three stages:

(i) by considering small displacements from the equilibrium point, we replace equation (7.17) by the linear equations (7.20);

(ii) we eliminate one of the variables, to reach equation (7.21);

(iii) the solution of (7.21) is given in appendix 4; we therefore examine this solution to see whether it describes an oscillation.

First, we consider small displacements from the equilibrium concentrations, Y_E and Z_E. Since at equilibrium $dY/dt = dZ/dt = 0$, we have

$$\left.\begin{array}{r}\dfrac{c}{a+lZ_E} - kY_E = 0, \\[2mm] eY_E - fZ_E = 0.\end{array}\right\} \qquad (7.18)$$

Z_E can easily be eliminated, giving a quadratic equation for Y_E. Fortunately, however there is no need to solve equations (7.18) to discover the behaviour of (7.17).

Thus let $\qquad\qquad Y = Y_E + y; \quad Z = Z_E + z.$

Then $\qquad \dfrac{dY}{dt} = \dfrac{dy}{dt} = \dfrac{c}{a+lZ_E+lz} - kY_E - ky.$

The right-hand side of this equation would be greatly simplified if it could be expressed in the form

$$\frac{c}{a+lZ_E} + \phi(z) - kY_E - ky = \phi(z) - ky,$$

always provided, of course, that $\phi(z)$ turns out to be not too complicated. We therefore proceed (see appendix 6) as follows:

$$\frac{c}{a+lZ_E+lz} = \frac{c}{a+lZ_E} \times \frac{a+lZ_E}{a+lZ_E+lz}$$

$$= \frac{c}{a+lZ_E} \div \frac{a+lZ_E+lz}{a+lZ_E}$$

$$= \frac{c}{a+lZ_E}\left\{1 + \frac{lz}{a+lZ_E}\right\}^{-1}$$

and since when z is small, $(1+Rz)^{-1} \simeq 1 - Rz$,

$$\frac{c}{a+lZ_E+lz} = \frac{c}{a+lZ_E}\left\{1 - \frac{lz}{a+lZ_E}\right\}$$

and hence $\qquad \left.\begin{array}{l}\dfrac{dy}{dt} = -\dfrac{clz}{(a+lZ_E)^2} - ky \\[4mm] \dfrac{dz}{dt} = ey - fz.\end{array}\right\} \qquad (7.19)$

and

Equations (7.19) can be written:

$$dy/dt = -Kz - ky, \quad dz/dt = ey - fz, \qquad (7.20)$$

where K, k, e and f are all positive.

We now proceed to the second stage, to eliminate one of the variables. To do this, we differentiate both sides of the first equation:

$$\frac{d^2y}{dt^2} = -K\frac{dz}{dt} - k\frac{dy}{dt}.$$

Substituting for dz/dt from (7.20), this becomes

$$\frac{d^2y}{dt^2} = -K(ey - fz) - k\frac{dy}{dt},$$

and if we now substitute, from (7.20),

$$z = -\frac{1}{K}\left(\frac{dy}{dt} + ky\right),$$

and then collect terms, we get

$$\frac{d^2y}{dt^2} + (f+k)\frac{dy}{dt} + (fk + Ke)y = 0. \qquad (7.21)$$

From appendix 4, the solution of this equation is of the form

$$y = \alpha e^{\lambda_1 t} + \beta e^{\lambda_2 t},$$

where

$$\lambda_1, \lambda_2 = \frac{-(f+k) \pm \sqrt{[(f+k)^2 - 4(fk + Ke)]}}{2}$$

$$= \frac{-(f+k) \pm \sqrt{[(f-k)^2 - 4Ke]}}{2}.$$

If the expression under the square root sign is negative, this describes a damped oscillation, since $-(f+k)$ is negative. If the expression under the square root is positive, then since

$$(f+k) > +\sqrt{[(f-k)^2 - 4Ke]},$$

as must be the case when all the constants are positive, both λ_1 and λ_2 are negative, and the system does not oscillate.

Thus a control system of this kind is either non-oscillating, or leads to a damped oscillation. However a slight modification of these equations, which allows for the fact that a certain time necessarily elapses while mRNA molecules travel from the gene locus to the ribosome, gives rise to an oscillatory system.

The delay introduced because mRNA must travel from nucleus to ribosome can approximately be allowed for as follows. Instead of equations (7.14–16) we write:

$$\left. \begin{aligned} \frac{dY}{dt} &= \frac{c}{a+bM} - kY, \\[1em] \frac{dZ}{dt} &= e\,Y_{t-T} - fZ, \\[1em] \frac{dM}{dt} &= gZ - hM. \end{aligned} \right\} \qquad (7.22)$$

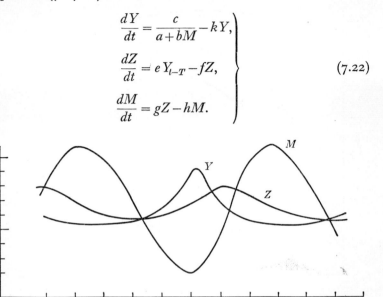

Fig. 31. Computer solution of equations (7.22). Y is the nuclear concentration of mRNA, Z the cytoplasmic concentration, and M the enzyme concentration. (After Goodwin, B. C. G. (1965). *Advances in Enzymology*.)

In these equations Y is the concentration of mRNA in the nucleus at time t, and Y_{t-T} the concentration in the nucleus at time $t-T$. The only alteration which has been made to the equations is to assume that the rate of enzyme synthesis is proportional to the nuclear concentration of mRNA at time $(t-T)$. This is equivalent to assuming that the cytoplasmic concentration of mRNA resembles that in the nucleus T seconds earlier.

Equations (7.22) can be solved on a computer. The effect of introducing a delay of T seconds is to cause the system to oscillate. Fig. 31 shows the type of behaviour to be expected.

The figure shows that the amplitude does not change with time.

In fact if the system is started with a smaller amplitude than that shown, the amplitude increases with time; if with a larger amplitude, then the amplitude decreases with time. Such a system is said to reach a 'limit cycle'.

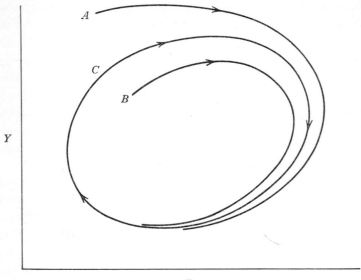

Fig. 32. The concepts of a phase space and a limit cycle. The state of the system described by equations (7.22) can be specified by the values of X, Y and Z; thus its state can be specified by a point in a 3-dimensional 'phase space'. In the figure, only two of these dimensions are shown. Knowing the state of the system, the equations tell us how it will change; the direction of change can be represented by trajectories in the phase space. For this particular system, if the system starts from a point on the loop C, it will continue to traverse this loop; i.e. it will oscillate with constant amplitude as shown in fig. 31. If it starts at a point outside (A) or inside (B) the loop, it will follow a spiral trajectory which approaches the 'limit cycle' C. (For clarity, the shape of the loop has been distorted so as to be more nearly circular.)

The reason for the phrase 'limit cycle' will be clearer if we plot the solution of equations (7.22) in a different way. Instead of plotting Y, Z and M against t, we will plot Y against Z, as in fig. 32. The closed loop represents an oscillation of constant amplitude, and the spiral trajectories indicate how the system will approach this loop, or 'limit cycle'.

Fig. 32 is an example of a 'phase diagram'. The state of the system at any instant can be described by specifying a number of variables— for example Y, the nuclear mRNA concentration and Z, the enzyme concentration. If two variables are adequate to describe the system, then its state can be described by a point in a plane; properly, we should also specify M, and so would require a 3-dimensional space in which to locate the state of the system. Such a space is called a 'phase space', which may have any number of dimensions. The future behaviour of the system can then be indicated by attaching to each point in the phase space an arrow, or 'vector', indicating the direction in which the system will move. By following these arrows, we can build up trajectories, and it is such trajectories which have been shown in fig. 32.

Another example of a phase diagram in this book is fig. 17; in that case, the state of the ecological system is specified by the abundance of two species. Similar diagrams have been widely used in population genetics to describe cases when genes are segregating at more than one locus; the state of the system is then specified by p_1, p_2, p_n, the frequencies of, say, the dominant allele at each of n loci. It is in fact often the case that the behaviour of a system can be presented in a more illuminating way in a phase diagram than by plotting the variables against time.

Examples

1 Devise a method of solving the equation

$$\frac{d^2x}{dt^2} + 2\frac{dx}{dt} + 3x = 0$$

by numerical iteration. If when $t = 0$, $x = 1$ and $dx/dt = 0$, find by numerical iteration the greatest negative value taken by x, and the time at which it is reached. Check these results by finding the analytical solution of the equation.

2 The forearm is to be moved rapidly by the contraction of the biceps through an angle of 30° from an initial stationary position to a 'goal' position. The moment of inertia of the forearm about the elbow is 5×10^5 gm-cm^2. The tendons of both the biceps muscle and its antagonist the triceps have constant moment arms, of 4 cms about the point of rotation of the elbow. The force P in grams exerted by the biceps at any moment is $2 \times 10^5 \theta$, where θ is the angle in radians between the actual position of the forearm and its goal position. The force R in grams in the triceps muscle is Kv, where v is the rate in cms/sec at which the triceps is increasing in length. If the arm swings past its goal, then the formulae for the forces P and R are interchanged.

(a) Find the values of K if (i) the movement is critically damped, (ii) the arm overshoots its goal by $3°$.

(b) Find, by plotting graphs of θ against time, the time taken for the limb to reach a point within $3°$ of its goal in the two cases.

(c) A mass of 1 Kg is held in the hand, 30 cms from the elbow. If P and R obey the same equations as before, with K sufficient to give critical damping for the unloaded arm, by how much does the hand overshoot its goal?

Assume throughout that the movement occurs in a horizontal plane, so that the force of gravity can be ignored.

3 Two substances react accordingly to the formula $A + B \rightleftharpoons AB$, the concentrations being x_A, x_B and x_{AB}. The rate of the forward reaction is $Kx_A x_B$ and of the reverse reaction kx_{AB}. If initially x_{AB} is zero, and $x_A = A$, $x_B = B$, find an equation for dx_A/dt in terms of x_A, A, B, k and K.

Readers familiar with the method of integrating $1/(a + bx + cx^2)$ can solve this equation and satisfy themselves that it is non-oscillatory.

4 Modify equations (7.17) on the assumption that mRNA and enzyme are removed at a constant rate, independant of their concentrations. Show that for small displacements from the equilibrium the system oscillates with a period $\dfrac{2\pi}{k} \sqrt{\dfrac{c}{le}}$.

5 Sketch approximately a phase diagram of the behaviour of the predator–prey system described by equations (3.7 and 3.8) when $R = r = 2$ and $CX_E = 1$.

8 DIFFUSION AND SIMILAR PROCESSES

A. The notation of 'partial differentiation'

This chapter, instead of discussing a single biological topic, introduces a new mathematical notation, that of 'partial differentiation', which is useful in a number of different fields of biology. So far, the equations we have considered describe the behaviour of one or more 'dependent variables'—e.g. the frequencies of genes, or the length of a muscle—as functions of a single 'independent variable', which has usually been time. There is however a class of problem in which we want to talk about the behaviour of a dependent variable as a function of two or more independent variables. Such a treatment leads to partial differential equations.

Unfortunately, to find analytical solutions to such equations usually calls for mathematical techniques beyond those which have been assumed in readers of this book. Nevertheless, a familiarity with the notation enables one to follow other people's arguments, even if one could not have developed the argument oneself. It is for this reason that the present chapter is included.

An example to illustrate the notation is shown in fig. 33. This shows a hill, whose height above sea level is given by

$$h = y \sin x, \tag{8.1}$$

where x is the distance in an easterly direction from point O, and y the distance in a northerly direction.

Consider a man walking due east along a line which passes a distance y_1 north of O. At any moment his height is $h = y_1 \sin x$, and his path has a slope

$$\frac{dh}{dx} = y_1 \cos x. \tag{8.2}$$

It is convenient to have a short way of writing this slope—i.e. the rate of change of h relative to x, while y is held constant. In fact we write this 'partial differential' of h relative to x as

$$\frac{\partial h}{\partial x} = y \cos x, \qquad (8.3)$$

and similarly, the rate of change of h relative to y, while x is held constant, is written

$$\frac{\partial h}{\partial y} = \sin x. \qquad (8.4)$$

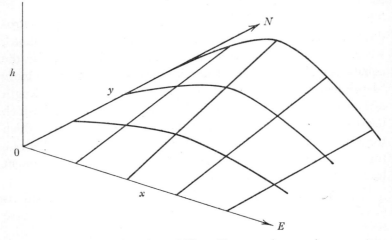

Fig. 33. An imaginary hill, to illustrate the notation
of partial differentiation.

Thus in deriving (8.3) from (8.1) we differentiate $y \sin x$ with respect to x, assuming y is constant, and in deriving (8.4) we differentiate with respect to y, assuming x is constant.

In this example, both the independent variables x and y are distances. In the examples discussed later in this chapter, one of the independent variables is a distance and one is time. We shall therefore be describing the behaviour of a dependant variable which varies in space and time. As an example, fig. 34 shows the height h of a skipping rope above the ground, as a function of the time t, and of the horizontal distance s from one end of the rope. $\partial h/\partial s$ then refers to the slope of the rope relative to the ground at any instant of time, and $\partial h/\partial t$ to the vertical component of velocity of a fixed point on the rope.

Thus if, as will be approximately the case,

$$h = \sin \alpha s \cos \beta t,$$

then $\quad \partial h/\partial s = \alpha \cos \alpha s \cos \beta t; \quad \partial h/\partial t = -\beta \sin \alpha s \sin \beta t.$

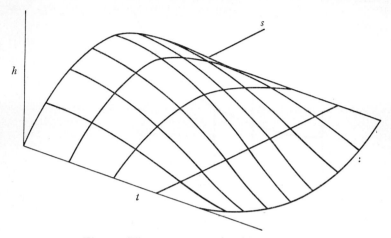

Fig. 34. The movement of a skipping rope.

B. Diffusion

The first problem to which this notation will be applied is that of diffusion along a tube. Fig. 35 shows the concentration x of some substance plotted against s, the distance along the tube. If the cross-sectional area of the tube is a, there is an amount ax of the substance per unit length of the tube, and hence the amount in a short length δs of the tube is $ax\,\delta s$.

The rate at which the amount of substance in element δs is increasing is $A - B$, where A and B are the rates of diffusion from left to right across the two faces of the element.

Thus

$$\frac{\partial}{\partial t}(ax\,\delta s) = a\,\delta s \cdot \frac{\partial x}{\partial t} = A - B. \tag{8.5}$$

Now the rate at which a substance diffuses across a surface is proportional to the area of the surface, and to the concentration gradient at right-angles to the surface.

Hence $\quad A = -a\mu\left(\dfrac{\partial x}{\partial s}\right)$ at s; $\quad B = -a\mu\left(\dfrac{\partial x}{\partial s}\right)$ at $s+\delta s$;

where μ is a constant depending on the temperature and the substance diffusing, and the minus sign arises because when $\partial x/\partial s$ is positive, diffusion would be from right to left, and so A and B would be negative.

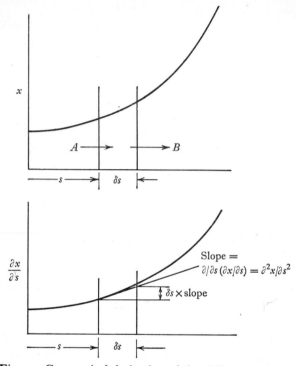

Fig. 35. Geometrical derivation of the diffusion equation.

Hence
$$A - B = -a\mu\left[\left(\frac{\partial x}{\partial s}\right) \text{ at } s - \left(\frac{\partial x}{\partial s}\right) \text{ at } s+\delta s\right],$$

and as is shown diagrammatically in fig. 35, the expression in the square bracket is equal to $-\delta s \cdot \partial^2 x/\partial s^2$.

And so substituting in (8.5)

$$\frac{\partial x}{\partial t} = \mu\frac{\partial^2 x}{\partial s^2}, \tag{8.6}$$

which is a partial differential equation describing diffusion along a tube. The equation can be seen to make sense; it says that if the graph of x against s is concave upwards, then x is increasing at this point, and *vice-versa*.

Equation (8.6) has an analytical solution, but it is rather tricky to find. However, we can answer some of the interesting questions about diffusion without finding a general solution.

Consider first the case of a tube of length l and cross-sectional area a connecting two large reservoirs, which are maintained at different concentrations X_0 and X_1. When a steady state has been reached, how rapidly will substances pass along the tube, and in particular, how will this vary with l? This is equivalent to the case when two solutions are separated by a layer of tissue of thickness l and area a.

When a steady state has been reached, $\partial x/\partial t = 0$; i.e. at any point along the tube the concentration does not vary with time. Hence from (8.6)

$$\frac{\partial^2 x}{\partial s^2} = 0.$$

Therefore $x = cs + d$, where c and d are constants. When $s = 0$, $x = X_0$, and when $s = l$, $x = X_1$, and hence

$$X_0 = d; \; X_1 = cl + d$$

$$= cl + X_0$$

$$\therefore \quad c = \frac{1}{l}(X_1 - X_0)$$

and so

$$x = X_0 - \frac{(X_0 - X_1)s}{l}. \tag{8.7}$$

This solution is shown in fig. 36. It shows that the concentration gradient is a straight line with a slope of $-(X_0 - X_1)/l$. Hence the rate of diffusion along the tube is equal to

$$a(X_0 - X_1)/l$$

and in particular is inversely proportional to the length of the tube.

Consider now the situation before a steady state is reached. Suppose that a tube is connected to a reservoir whose concentration is maintained at X_0, and that at time $t = 0$ the concentration in the tube is zero. How long will it take for the concentration at some point along the tube to reach a particular value? i.e. if a concentration $kX_0 (k < 1)$ is reached at a distance l along the tube at time T, how will T vary with l?

We can guess the answer to this question by looking at fig. 37, which shows the concentration x at time T, when a concentration kX_0 has been reached at a distance l. The following guesses seem plausible:

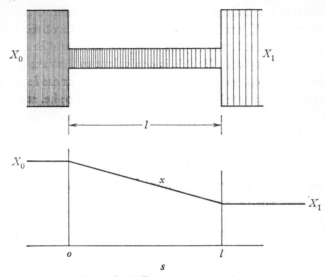

Fig. 36. Diffusion along a tube.

(i) The amount of substance which must diffuse from the reservoir into the tube in time T is equal to the area under the curve in fig. 37, and this is proportional to l.

(ii) The rate at which substance diffuses into the tube is proportional to the gradient at $s = 0$, and at time T this gradient is proportional to $1/l$. The average rate at which substance has entered the tube during the interval $t = 0$ to $t = T$ may likewise be proportional to $1/l$.

If these guesses are right, then

$$T \propto l \div 1/l \quad \text{or} \quad T \propto l^2.$$

In words, the time taken for a particular concentration to be reached is proportional to the square of the distance. The conjecture is confirmed by an analytical solution of (8.6).

c. Morphogenesis; the development of patterns

Equation (8.6) is perhaps not very interesting, since nothing emerges from it which cannot be seen, at least qualitatively, without getting involved in partial differentials. However, if we allow simultaneously for the effects of diffusion and chemical reaction, some unexpected results emerge.

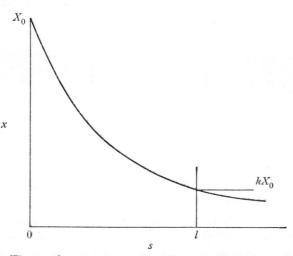

Fig. 37. Concentration of a diffusing substance along
a tube before a steady state is reached.

Let the concentrations of two chemical substances, A and B, in solution in a tube be X and Y. We are interested in changes in X and Y as functions of the time t and of the distance s along the tube.

Consider first changes in X and Y due to chemical reactions. We suppose that substrates from which A and B can be synthesised and to which they can be degraded, and also the relevant enzymes, are present. There will then be some values of the concentrations X_E and Y_E for which there is a chemical equilibrium. As on many occasions before, we write

$$X = X_E + x; \quad Y = Y_E + y,$$

so that x and y measure the departures of the concentrations from their equilibrium values.

Now when $x = y = 0$, then $\partial x/\partial t = \partial y/\partial t = 0$. Hence for small displacements from the equilibrium, we have

$$\partial x/\partial t = ax + by; \quad \partial y/\partial t = cx + dy,$$

where a, b, c and d are constants.

Allowing also for diffusion along the tube, if μ and ν are constants describing the rates of diffusion of A and B respectively, then

$$\left.\begin{aligned}
\frac{\partial x}{\partial t} &= ax + by + \mu\,\frac{\partial^2 x}{\partial s^2}, \\
\frac{\partial y}{\partial t} &= cx + dy + \nu\,\frac{\partial^2 y}{\partial s^2}.
\end{aligned}\right\} \tag{8.8}$$

These equations were first obtained by Turing (*Phil. Trans.* B **237**, 37). They have an analytical solution, but the methods of reaching it are complicated. However, the interesting features of their behaviour can be illustrated graphically.

Clearly, if at time $t = 0$, x and y are zero for all values of s (i.e. all along the tube), then $\partial x/\partial t = \partial y/\partial t = 0$, so that x and y continue to be zero. We are interested in the behaviour of the system if this homogeneous equilibrium is disturbed. As we would expect, the usual answer is that the equilibrium is restored; i.e. for most values of the reaction rates a, b, c, and d and the diffusion rates μ and ν, as t increases x and y tend to zero everywhere.

Surprisingly, however, there are values of the constants for which the homogeneous equilibrium is unstable. In such cases, even if the system starts in a homogeneous state, with $x = y = 0$ everywhere, a 'standing wave' of concentration of the morphogens may arise from any small initial disturbance. It is quite easy to see how this can happen without solving the equations.

Thus we will make the following assumptions:

(1) a and c are positive—i.e. if the concentration of A rises above its equilibrium level, the rate of synthesis of both A and B rises.

(2) b is negative—i.e. if the concentration of B rises, it leads to destruction of A. (d can be assumed to be zero.)

(3) $\nu > \mu$—i.e. B diffuses faster than A.

Fig. 38 shows what will happen. In fig. 38 *a* it is supposed that the homogeneous equilibrium is disturbed by a small local rise in the concentration of *A*. In fig. 38 *b* this has led to a further rise in *A* and a rise in *B*, but *B* has diffused out further. At the point marked by an arrow, *y* is positive and *x* zero, so that there is a net destruction of *A*, leading to the condition shown in fig. 38 *c*. This will in turn

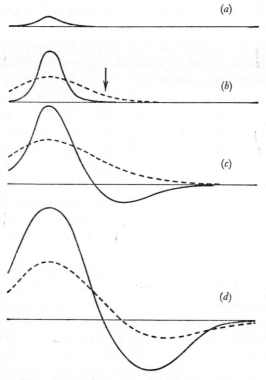

Fig. 38. Development of a standing wave.

lead to destruction of morphogen *B*, so that a 'trough' will develop on either side of the initial 'peak' (fig. 38 *d*). These troughs will cause the development of further peaks, and so on until a standing wave has developed, whose 'chemical wave-length' will depend on the values of the constants defining the rates of reaction and diffusion.

This result can be seen to be true by graphical methods, but would hardly have been discovered by such means in the first place. Its possible relevance to biology lies in the field of morphogenesis, and in particular in the development of regular patterns of repeated parts such as bristles in *Drosophila*, feather papillae in birds or stomata in plants. If the tube is replaced by a strip of tissue, and if one of the substances A and B has the effect, if its concentration rises above some threshold level, of inducing cells in that region to differentiate in a particular way, then we have a mechanism for the regular spacing of structures in an initially homogeneous field.

Phenomena similar to those of diffusion arise in other branches of biology. To give two examples:

(i) In ecology, what are the consequences for population regulation of the fact that animals move about? If in any given region conditions give rise to a density fluctuation, to what extent will movements of individuals synchronise such fluctuations over a wide area? If conditions vary from place to place, will movement tend to damp out oscillations which would otherwise take place?

Such problems have been little studied, perhaps because the equations are intractable. However, the development of computers has removed this objection, and this would now seem to be a promising field for research.

(ii) Epidemics such as Asian flu appear to travel like a wave across the earth. A promising start has been made on the mathematical analysis of this process. The treatment requires partial differential equations because we want to describe changes in P, the proportion of people having flu, as a function of time t and distance s.

APPENDICES

Appendix 1: Exponential and logarithmic functions

We start by defining a function of x, $\exp(x)$, by an infinite series:

$$\exp(x) = 1 + x + \frac{x^2}{2!} + \frac{x^3}{3!} + \ldots + \frac{x^n}{n!} + \ldots \tag{1}$$

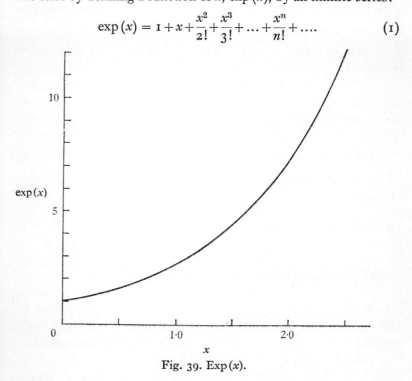

Fig. 39. Exp (x).

It can be shown that this series converges (i.e. has a finite sum) for all values of x. This series was chosen because, as can easily be verified,

$$\frac{d}{dx}\exp(x) = \exp(x). \tag{2}$$

In fig. 39 $\exp(x)$ is shown plotted against x; it is a graph whose slope is equal to its height above the x axis.

The value of $\exp(x)$ when $x = 1$ is a number called e. Thus $e = 1 + 1 + \dfrac{1}{2!} + \dfrac{1}{3!} + \dots$. By summing terms it can be calculated that $e \simeq 2 \cdot 718$.

We will now prove that $\exp(x) = e^x$. The first step is to prove that $\exp(x) \times \exp(y) = \exp(x+y)$. To multiply together two infinite series sounds a more complicated undertaking than it in fact is. The product clearly consists of a number of terms of the form $kx^a y^b$. We collect together all the terms in which $a + b = n$, as follows:

$$\frac{x^n}{n!} + \frac{x^{n-1}y}{(n-1)!} + \dots + \frac{x^{n-r}y^r}{(n-r)!\,r!} + \dots + \frac{y^n}{n!}$$

$$= \frac{1}{n!}\left\{ x^n + nx^{n-1}y + \dots + \frac{n!}{(n-r)!\,r!}x^{n-r}y^r + \dots + y^n \right\}$$

$$= \frac{(x+y)^n}{n!} \quad \text{which is a typical term of } \exp(x+y).$$

Hence $\qquad \exp(x) \times \exp(y) = \exp(x+y) \dots \qquad (3)$

By repeated application of (3), it follows that if n is any positive integer,

$$[\exp(x)]^n = \exp(nx),$$

and when $x = 1$, this becomes

$$\exp(n) = [\exp(1)]^n = e^n.$$

We have therefore proved the theorem

$$\exp(x) = e^x \qquad (4)$$

for the particular case when x is a positive integer. It is fairly easy to extend this proof to cover the case when x is a rational number— i.e. when $x = a/b$, and a and b are integers.

When x is a rational number, a/b, we know what e^x means: e^x means $\sqrt[b]{e^a}$—i.e. the number which multiplied by itself b times equals e^a. But if x an irrational number (i.e. one which cannot be expressed as a fraction—e.g. $\sqrt{2}$ or π) this definition will not do; how would you multiply a number by itself $\sqrt{2}$ times? We therefore *define* e^x, when x is irrational, by the series (1); thus we do not have to prove (4) for irrational numbers, because we have made it true by definition.

We now *define* 'natural logarithms' as follows: if $y = e^x$, then x is the natural logarithm of y. We write this as $x = \ln y$. In other words, natural logarithms are logarithms to the base e.

It is convenient to be able to convert natural logarithms into logarithms to the base 10.

Suppose $e^\alpha = 10$. Then by numerical calculation based on (1), it can be found that $\alpha \simeq 2\cdot303$. Now if $e^\alpha = 10$, then

$$e^{\alpha x} = 10^x = y \quad \text{say.}$$

Then $\qquad\qquad x = \log_{10} y \quad \text{and} \quad \alpha x = \ln y.$

Hence $\qquad\qquad \ln y = \alpha \log_{10} y,$

and so the conversion from natural logarithms is made by

$$\ln y \simeq 2\cdot303 \log_{10} y. \tag{5}$$

Notice that $e^0 = \exp(0) = 1$ from series (1), and hence $\ln 1 = 0$. Returning now to (2), we have, if $x = e^z$, then

$$dx/dz = e^z = x.$$

Hence $\qquad\qquad \int \frac{1}{x} dx = \int dz = A + z = A + \ln x,$

where A is the constant of integration. Thus we have now found the integral of x^{-1}. Ignoring arbitrary constants,

$$\int x^{-1} dx = \ln x. \tag{6}$$

It is sometimes convenient to express $\ln(1+x)$ as an infinite series. Thus

$$\ln(1+x) = \int (1+x)^{-1} dx,$$

and provided that x lies between -1 and $+1$, we can expand $(1+x)^{-1}$ by the binomial theorem, and hence

$$\ln(1+x) = \int (1 - x + x^2 - x^3 + \dots) dx.$$

If $x < 1$, the terms in this series get successively smaller, and it can be proved that the series has a finite sum. With this proviso, it is reasonable to integrate the series term by term, giving

$$\ln(1+x) = x - \tfrac{1}{2}x^2 + \tfrac{1}{3}x^3 - \tfrac{1}{4}x^4 + \dots$$

when $-1 < x < 1$.

Summarising, we *define*

$$\exp(x) = 1 + x + x^2/2! + \dots + x^n/n! + \dots$$

and $$e = \exp(1) = 1 + 1 + 1/2! + \dots \simeq 2{\cdot}718,$$

and we then prove that

$$\exp(x) = e^x \quad \text{and} \quad de^x/dx = e^x.$$

If $y = e^x$, we *define* $x = \ln y$.

We then show that

$$\ln y \simeq 2{\cdot}303 \log_{10} y \quad \text{and} \quad \int x^{-1}\,dx = \ln x.$$

Appendix 2: The circular functions, $\sin x$ and $\cos x$

In many ways, it would be convenient to start by defining $\sin x$ and $\cos x$ by infinite series, as we did $\exp x$, and then to derive their other properties from these series. However, most people first meet $\sin x$ in elementary trigonometry, to mean 'perpendicular/hypotenuse', and $\cos x$ to mean 'base/hypotenuse'. Starting from these geometrical definitions, it can be shown that:

(i) if x is measured in radians, then when x is small $\sin x \simeq x$ and $\cos x \simeq 1$.

(ii) $\dfrac{d}{dx}\sin x = \cos x$ and $\dfrac{d}{dx}\cos x = -\sin x$.

Hence $\dfrac{d^2}{dx^2}\sin x = -\sin x$ and $\dfrac{d^2}{dx^2}\cos x = -\cos x$.

We will now find infinite series which have these properties. We first seek a series for the function $\phi(x)$ such that $d^2\phi(x)/dx^2 = -\phi(x)$.

Let $$\phi(x) = a + bx + cx^2 + dx^3 + ex^4 + \dots.$$

Then $$d^2\phi(x)/dx^2 = 2c + 3.2.dx + 4.3ex^2 + \dots$$

and hence $$c = -\tfrac{1}{2}a; \quad e = -\frac{c}{4.3}; \quad g = -\frac{e}{6.5}\dots$$

and $$d = -\frac{b}{3\cdot 2}; \quad f = -\frac{d}{5\cdot 4} \quad \text{and so on.}$$

Hence $$\phi(x) = a\left(1 - \frac{x^2}{2!} + \frac{x^4}{4!} - \frac{x^6}{6!} + \ldots\right)$$
$$+ b\left(x - \frac{x^3}{3!} + \frac{x^5}{5!} - \frac{x^7}{7!} + \ldots\right).$$

Thus both the series in brackets satisfy the condition that $d^2\phi(x)/dx^2 = -\phi(x)$. By condition (i) above, it is clear that

$$\sin x = x - \frac{x^3}{3!} + \frac{x^5}{5!} - \frac{x^7}{7!} + \ldots, \qquad (7)$$

and $$\cos x = 1 - \frac{x^2}{2!} + \frac{x^4}{4!} - \frac{x^6}{6!} + \ldots. \qquad (8)$$

Appendix 3: Complex numbers

The necessity to invent a new kind of number arises because many equations commonly met with have no solution if we are restricted to the ordinary, so-called 'real', numbers. Thus the equation

$$x^2 + 2x + 3 = 0$$

has no real solution. Applying the usual formula for the solution of quadratic equations gives

$$x = \frac{-2 \pm \sqrt{(4-12)}}{2} = -1 \pm \sqrt{-2},$$

and negative numbers have no real square roots.

We get over this difficulty by defining $i = \sqrt{-1}$; that is, i is a number which, if multiplied by itself, gives -1. When first met with, this device inevitably arouses discomfort and even distrust. An attempt will be made in a moment to allay this distrust by giving a geometrical interpretation of i. But first, how are we going to operate with i, and how is it going to help us?

First, note that if $i^2 = -1$, then $i^3 = i^2 \times i = -i$, $i^4 = i^2 \times i^2 = +1$, and so on, and that $1/i = i/i^2 = i/-1 = -i$.

Returning to the equation that we started with, we note that $\sqrt{-2} = \sqrt{(-1 \times 2)} = i\sqrt{2}$, so that a solution of the equation is

$$x = -1 + i\sqrt{2}.$$

A number of this kind is called a 'complex' number. The symbol z is often used for complex numbers. A typical complex number $z = x + iy$ has a 'real' part x, and an 'imaginary' part iy.

Complex numbers are added and multiplied according to the usual rules of algebra. Thus if

$$z_1 = x_1 + iy_1; \quad z_2 = x_2 + iy_2.$$

Then
$$z_1 + z_2 = (x_1 + x_2) + i(y_1, + y_2),$$

and
$$z_1 \times z_2 = (x_1 + iy_1)(x_2 + iy_2)$$

$$= x_1 x_2 + ix_1 y_2 + ix_2 y_1 + i^2 y_1 y_2$$

$$= (x_1 x_2 - y_1 y_2) + i(x_1 y_2 + x_2 y_1).$$

Further, if two complex numbers are equal, both their real and imaginary parts are equal. Thus if $z_1 = z_2$, then $x_1 = x_2$ and $y_1 = y_2$.

Using these rules for addition and multiplication, you should satisfy yourself that $x = -1 + i\sqrt{2}$ is in fact a solution of the equation $x^2 + 2x + 3 = 0$.

An attempt will now be made to allay some of the reader's natural misgivings about this procedure. We are accustomed to the idea that all real numbers can be arranged along a line, positive numbers conventionally to the right of the origin and negative numbers to the left. I think that much of our initial discomfort about imaginary numbers arises from a well-founded conviction that there is no room for i along this line. My own difficulties largely disappeared when a geometrical method of representing complex numbers was shown to me.

A real number, e.g. $+4$, can be represented by a vector as in fig. 40. This vector could be converted into the vector -4 by rotating it through $180°$; it is conventional to rotate anti-clockwise. Hence since $-4 = +4 \times (-1)$, the operation $\times (-1)$ is equivalent to 'rotate anti-clockwise through $180°$'. Now the operation $\times i$ is one which, if performed twice, is equivalent to $\times (-1)$. Thus we can interpret $\times i$ as 'rotate through $90°$', as in fig. 40.

A complex number $z = x + iy$ can now be interpreted as a point in a plane, as in fig. 41. Such a representation is called an 'Argand diagram'. To convince yourself that this geometrical interpretation

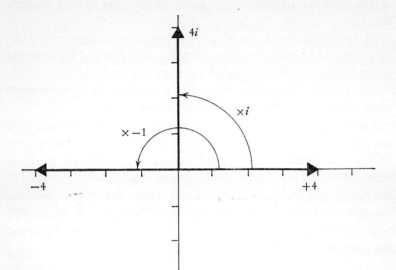

Fig. 40. Vector representation of $\times -1$ and $\times i$.

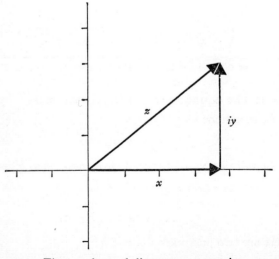

Fig. 41. Argand diagram; $z = x + iy$.

agrees with the algebraic rules given earlier, you should confirm that:

(i) the algebraic rule for addition given above corresponds to the geometrical process of 'vector addition', as performed for example when adding forces by a 'parallelogram of forces'; and

(ii) if $z = x + iy$, then the algebraic value of $iz = ix - y$ is properly represented by rotating the vector z through $90°$.

These geometrical representations are not used in this book; they are given in the hope that they will encourage the reader to operate with greater confidence. Our need for complex numbers in the book arises because a number of the equations studied have solutions of the form $x = A\lambda^n$, or $x = A e^{\lambda t}$, where λ is the solution of a quadratic equation, and may therefore be complex. The equations which lead to these solutions are discussed in appendices 4 and 5. We there use the identity

$$e^{ix} = \cos x + i \sin x, \tag{9}$$

which we will now prove. The proof follows directly from the series for e^x, $\sin x$ and $\cos x$. Thus

$$e^{ix} = 1 + ix - \frac{x^2}{2!} - i\frac{x^3}{3!} + \frac{x^4}{4!} + i\frac{x^5}{5!} - \dots$$

$$= \left(1 - \frac{x^2}{2!} + \frac{x^4}{4!} - \dots\right) + i\left(x - \frac{x^3}{3!} + \frac{x^5}{5!} - \dots\right)$$

$$= \cos x + i \sin x \quad \text{as stated above.}$$

Appendix 4: The equation $x_{n+2} + b x_{n+1} + c x_n = 0$

To solve the equation:

$$x_{n+2} + b x_{n+1} + c x_n = 0 \tag{10}$$

we guess the solution $x_n = A\lambda^n$. Substituting in (10) gives

$$A\lambda^{n+2} + Ab\lambda^{n+1} + Ac\lambda^n = 0,$$

$$\therefore \quad \lambda^2 + b\lambda + c = 0.$$

Hence there are two possible values of λ:

$$\lambda_1 = -\frac{b}{2} + \frac{\sqrt{(b^2 - 4c)}}{2}; \quad \lambda_2 = -\frac{b}{2} - \frac{\sqrt{(b^2 - 4c)}}{2},$$

and the complete solution of (10) is

$$x_n = A\lambda_1^n + B\lambda_2^n, \tag{11}$$

where A and B are constants which can be chosen to fit the initial conditions.

If $b^2 - 4c$ is positive, this form of solution is satisfactory. But if $b^2 - 4c$ is negative, λ_1 and λ_2 are complex, and we need to express (11) in a different form. To do this, we use equation (9), appendix 3:

$$e^{i\theta} = \cos\theta + i\sin\theta,$$

and hence $\qquad e^{in\theta} = \cos n\theta + i\sin n\theta.$

Thus if λ_1 is complex, we write $\lambda_1 = De^{i\theta}$, and find D and θ as follows:

$$De^{i\theta} = D\cos\theta + Di\sin\theta = -\frac{b}{2} + i\frac{\surd(4c-b^2)}{2}.$$

If this equation is to be satisfied, both real and imaginary parts must balance, and so

$$D\cos\theta = -\frac{b}{2}, \qquad \therefore \; D^2\cos^2\theta = \frac{b^2}{4}$$

$$D\sin\theta = \frac{\surd(4c-b^2)}{2}, \quad \therefore \; D^2\sin^2\theta = \frac{4c-b^2}{4}$$

hence, adding: $\qquad\qquad\qquad\overline{D^2 \qquad\quad = c}$

$$\therefore \quad D \quad\;\; = \surd c$$

and $\qquad\qquad \cos\theta = -\frac{b}{2D} = -\frac{b}{2\surd c}.$

Similarly, if we write $\lambda_2 = Ee^{i\phi}$, we find

$$E\cos\phi = -\frac{b}{2}; \quad E\sin\phi = -\frac{\surd(4c-b^2)}{2}.$$

Whence $E = \surd c = D$, and

$$\cos\phi = \cos\theta, \quad \sin\phi = -\sin\theta,$$

and these conditions are satisfied if $\phi = 2\pi - \theta$.

Hence

$$x_n = AD^n e^{in\theta} + BE^n e^{in\phi}$$
$$= D^n\{A[\cos n\theta + i\sin n\theta] + B[\cos n(2\pi-\theta) + i\sin n(2\pi-\theta)]\},$$

and since

$$\cos n(2\pi - \theta) = \cos n\theta; \quad \sin n(2\pi - \theta) = -\sin n\theta,$$
$$x_n = D^n\{(A+B)\cos n\theta + (A-B)\,i\sin n\theta\}.$$

A and B are arbitrary constants. In practical problems, x_n is always real, and hence $(A+B)$ must be a real number and $(A-B)$ an imaginary number. This of course requires that A and B be complex numbers.

If
$$A = \tfrac{1}{2}(k_1 - k_2 i); \quad B = \tfrac{1}{2}(k_1 + k_2 i),$$

then
$$A + B = k_1; \quad A - B = -k_2 i,$$

and hence
$$x_n = D^n(k_1 \cos n\theta + k_2 \sin n\theta) \tag{12}$$

where
$$D = \sqrt{c} \quad \text{and} \quad \theta = \cos^{-1}\left(-\frac{b}{2\sqrt{c}}\right),$$

and k_1 and k_2 can be chosen to satisfy the initial conditions.

(12) is the alternative form of (11) we have been seeking. It describes an oscillation, which increases in amplitude if $D = \sqrt{c} > 1$, and which is damped if $\sqrt{c} < 1$.

Summarising:

(i) if $b^2 > 4c$, there are no oscillations. (11) describes the behaviour of x, which increases without limit if $\lambda_1 > 1$;

(ii) if $b^2 < 4c$, x oscillates, with an amplitude which increases with time if $c > 1$.

Appendix 5: The equation $\dfrac{d^2x}{dt^2} + b\dfrac{dx}{dt} + cx = 0$

To solve the equation:

$$\frac{d^2x}{dt^2} + b\frac{dx}{dt} + cx = 0 \tag{13}$$

we guess the solution $x = A\,e^{\lambda t}$. Substituting this in (13) gives

$$A\lambda^2 e^{\lambda t} + Ab\lambda e^{\lambda t} + Ac\,e^{\lambda t} = 0,$$

$$\therefore \quad \lambda^2 + b\lambda + c = 0,$$

an equation which has two solutions,

$$\lambda_1 = -\frac{b}{2} + \frac{\sqrt{(b^2 - 4c)}}{2}; \quad \lambda_2 = -\frac{b}{2} - \frac{\sqrt{(b^2 - 4c)}}{2}.$$

Thus $x = A\,e^{\lambda_1 t}$ and $x = B\,e^{\lambda_2 t}$ are both solutions of (13), whatever the value of the constants A and B. It is easy to verify that

$$x = A\,e^{\lambda_1 t} + B\,e^{\lambda_2 t} \tag{14}$$

is also a solution; it is in fact the complete solution of (13).

If either λ_1 or λ_2 are positive, x will increase without limit with increasing t. Now if b is negative, λ_1 is necessarily positive (λ_2 will be positive too unless c is negative); if c is negative, λ_1 is necessarily positive. Hence if either b or c is negative, x will increase without limit.

But the interesting cases arise when both b and c are positive. There are two possibilities:

(i) $b^2 - 4c$ is positive. λ_1 and λ_2 are then both real and negative, and x decreases with increasing t, without oscillations.

(ii) $b^2 - 4c$ is negative. λ_1 and λ_2 are then complex numbers, and it is convenient to change the form of (14). For brevity, let

$$\frac{\sqrt{(4c - b^2)}}{2} = \alpha.$$

Then
$$x = A\,e^{(-\frac{1}{2}b + i\alpha)t} + B\,e^{(-\frac{1}{2}b - i\alpha)}$$

$$= e^{-\frac{1}{2}bt}(A\,e^{i\alpha t} + B\,e^{-i\alpha t}).$$

We now use equation (9), appendix 3,

$$e^{i\alpha t} = \cos \alpha t + i \sin \alpha t$$

and similarly
$$e^{-i\alpha t} = \cos(-\alpha t) + i \sin(-\alpha t)$$

$$= \cos \alpha t - i \sin \alpha t,$$

and hence
$$x = e^{-\frac{1}{2}bt}\{(A + B)\cos \alpha t + (A - B)\,i \sin \alpha t\}. \tag{15}$$

Since in actual problems x will be a real number, A and B must be chosen (cf. p. 136) so that $(A + B)$ is real and $(A - B)$ imaginary. If this is done, (15) can be rewritten

$$x = e^{-\frac{1}{2}bt}\left\{k_1 \cos \frac{\sqrt{(4c - b^2)}}{2}\,t + k_2 \sin \frac{\sqrt{(4c - b^2)}}{2}\,t\right\}, \tag{16}$$

where k_1 and k_2 are constants which can be chosen to fit the initial conditions.

Equation (16) describes an oscillation with a period $\dfrac{4\pi}{\sqrt{(4c-b^2)}}$, decreasing in amplitude with time provided that b is positive.

If b is zero, the equation

$$\frac{d^2x}{dt^2} + cx = 0$$

has the solution $x = k_1 \cos \sqrt{c}\, t + k_2 \sin \sqrt{c}\, t$, a harmonic oscillation with constant amplitude and period $2\pi/\sqrt{c}$.

Notice that in both (14) and (16) there are two arbitary constants, A and B in (14) and k_1 and k_2 in (16). This is the correct number of constants of integration for the solution of a 'second order' differential equation—i.e. for an equation in which the highest order differential is d^2y/dx^2.

Such an equation has to be integrated twice, so it is natural that there should be two constants. Perhaps a more convincing way of seeing that there ought to be two constants is as follows. Equation (13) can be regarded as giving the acceleration, d^2x/dt^2, in terms of the position, x, and velocity, dx/dt. A complete solution therefore is one which we can fit to any initial values of x and dx/dt, and this requires that there be two arbitrary constants.

A snag arises when the system is 'critically damped'. Thus suppose $b^2 = 4c$. Then $\lambda_1 = \lambda_2 = -b/2$, and (14) becomes

$$x = A\,e^{-bt/2}.$$

This cannot be the complete solution because it contains only one constant. It can be shown that when $b^2 = 4c$, $x = (A+Bt)\,e^{-bt/2}$ is a solution, whatever the values of A and B. We need not worry about the line of reasoning which leads to this solution; we can satisfy ourselves that it *is* a solution by finding dx/dt and d^2x/dt^2 and then substituting in (13), with $b^2 = 4c$.

Summarising:

(i)   if b or c is negative, x increases without limit;

(ii)   if b and c are positive, and b^2-4c is positive, then x decreases without oscillations;

(iii)   if $b^2 - 4c$ is negative, x oscillates, with decreasing amplitude provided that b is positive.

Appendix 6: How to reduce equations to a linear form

The equations considered in appendices 4 and 5 are called linear equations. It is usually possible to reduce finite difference and differential equations to a linear form if one is prepared to consider only small displacements from the equilibrium. This appendix lists some of the tricks which are useful in doing this. In all cases, a function of x is expanded in a power series, and it is then assumed that the terms in x^2, x^3 and so on can be neglected in comparison with the term in x.

(a) We can use the binomial expansion, according to which

$$(a+bx)^n = a^n + na^{n-1}bx + \frac{n(n-1)}{2!}a^{n-2}b^2x^2 + \dots.$$

Thus if x is small $\qquad (a+bx)^n \simeq a^n + na^{n-1}bx,$ \hfill (17)

and in particular

$$(1+x)^n \simeq 1+nx, \quad \sqrt{(1+x)} \simeq 1+\tfrac{1}{2}x$$

and

$$\frac{1}{(1+x)^n} \simeq 1-nx.$$

(b) Equation (17) holds if x is small, provided that n is not too large. But a look at the full binomial expansion shows that the terms in x^2, x^3, etc. are only negligible in comparison with the term in x if nx is small.

If x is small, but n large, so that nx is not small, we proceed as follows:

$$(1+x)^n = 1+nx + \frac{n(n-1)}{2!}x^2 + \frac{n(n-1)(n-2)}{3!}x^3 + \dots$$

and since when n is large, $nx \simeq (n-1)x \simeq (n-2)x$,

$$(1+x)^n \simeq 1+nx + \frac{n^2x^2}{2!} + \frac{n^3x^3}{3!} + \dots = e^{nx},$$

and similarly $\quad (a+bx)^n = a^n\left(1+\frac{bx}{a}\right)^n \simeq a^n e^{nbx/a}.$ \hfill (18)

(c) From the expansion in appendices 1 and 2, we have, when x is small: $\quad \sin x \simeq x, \quad \cos x \simeq 1, \quad e^x \simeq 1+x$

and $\qquad\qquad\qquad \ln(1+x) \simeq x.$

One final warning: if you are too enthusiastic in ignoring higher powers of x, you will sometimes finish up with the unhelpful equation, $o = o$. When this happens, there is nothing for it but to start again, taking into account the next highest power of x.

Appendix 7: Differentiation and integration

This appendix is intended as a reminder to those who have previously learnt how to differentiate and integrate.

A. *Differentiation*

(i) Definition:

$$\frac{d}{dx} f(x) = \lim_{\delta x \to 0} \frac{f(x + \delta x) - f(x)}{\delta x}.$$

This is equivalent to saying that the differential of $f(x)$ is the slope of the graph of $f(x)$ against x.

(ii) Standard differentials: by applying the definition given above, one can obtain the following table:

$f(x)$	$\frac{d}{dx} f(x)$
x^n	nx^{n-1}
$\sin ax$	$a \cos ax$
$\cos ax$	$-a \sin ax$
$\ln x$	$1/x$
e^{ax}	$a e^{ax}$

(iii) Methods of differentiation.

(*a*) Differentiation of a product:

$$\frac{d}{dx}(uv) = u \frac{dv}{dx} + v \frac{du}{dx}.$$

Hence for example $\dfrac{d}{dx} x \sin x = x \cos x + \sin x$.

(*b*) Differentiation of a quotient:

$$\frac{d}{dx} \frac{u}{v} = \frac{1}{v^2} \left\{ v \frac{du}{dx} - u \frac{dv}{dx} \right\}.$$

Hence for example:

$$\frac{d}{dx}\frac{\ln x}{x} = \frac{1}{x^2}\{x \times x^{-1} - \ln x\}$$

$$= \frac{1 - \ln x}{x^2}.$$

(c) Differentiation of a function of a function:

$$\frac{d}{dx}f(z) = \frac{df(z)}{dz}.\frac{dz}{dx}.$$

If you like to remember this by arguing that you could cancel the dzs, that is all right so long as you keep it to yourself.

Hence for example

$$\frac{d}{dx}\frac{1}{\sqrt{(1-x)}} = \frac{d}{d(1-x)}(1-x)^{-\frac{1}{2}}.\frac{d(1-x)}{dx},$$

$$= -\tfrac{1}{2}(1-x)^{-\frac{3}{2}} \times -1,$$

$$= \tfrac{1}{2}(1-x)^{-\frac{3}{2}};$$

and

$$\frac{d}{dx}\sin^3 x = \frac{d\sin^3 x}{d\sin x}.\frac{d\sin x}{dx},$$

$$= 3\sin^2 x \cos x.$$

B. *Integration*

(i) Definition.

If $\dfrac{d}{dx}f(x) = \phi(x)$ then $\displaystyle\int \phi(x)\,dx = f(x).$

i.e. we define integration as the opposite of differentiation. In general, we must include an arbitrary constant of integration, and write

$$\int \phi(x)\,dx = f(x) + C.$$

We can then define the definite integral

$$\int_a^b \phi(x)\,dx = f(b) - f(a).$$

It can be shown that this definite integral is equal to the area under the graph of $\phi(x)$ against x between $x = a$ and $x = b$.

(ii) Some standard integrals.

It is clear from the definition that the best way of integrating $\phi(x)$ is to know the answer; i.e. to know that $df(x)/dx = \phi(x)$. Using this method, we have:

$f(x)$	$\int f(x)\,dx$
x^n	$\dfrac{x^{n+1}}{n+1}$
$\sin ax$	$-\dfrac{1}{a}\cos ax$
$\cos ax$	$\dfrac{1}{a}\sin ax$
e^{ax}	$\dfrac{1}{a}e^{ax}$
x^{-1}	$\ln x$

(iii) Methods of integration.

(a) Substitution:

This is the most generally useful method of reducing a function to be integrated to one of the standard forms. For example, suppose we want to find

$$\int \frac{1}{\sqrt{(1-x)}}\,dx.$$

We might try the substitution

$$1 - x = z,$$

and hence

$$x = 1 - z,$$

$$\therefore \quad \frac{dx}{dz} = -1,$$

which we can write as $\quad dx = -dz.$

The justification for this rather odd procedure is given in sensible books on the calculus.

Hence

$$\int \frac{1}{\sqrt{(1-x)}}\,dx = -\int z^{-\frac{1}{2}}\,dz$$

$$= -2z^{\frac{1}{2}} = -2\sqrt{(1-x)}.$$

Sometimes it is not so easy to see what to substitute. For example

$$\int \frac{1}{\sqrt{(1-x^2)}} dx \quad \text{simplifies if we substitute} \quad x = \sin t.$$

Hence

$$\frac{dx}{dt} = \cos t \quad \text{and} \quad dx = \cos t \, dt.$$

Also

$$\sqrt{(1-x^2)} = \sqrt{(1-\sin^2 t)} = \cos t.$$

Hence

$$\int \frac{dx}{\sqrt{(1-x^2)}} = \int \frac{\cos t \, dt}{\cos t} = t = \sin^{-1} x.$$

Remember that when you substitute in a definite integral, the limits must be changed too. Thus

$$\int_0^1 \frac{dx}{\sqrt{(1-x^2)}} = \int_0^{\frac{1}{2}\pi} dt = [t]_0^{\frac{1}{2}\pi} = \tfrac{1}{2}\pi,$$

because, if

$$x = \sin t,$$

when

$$x = 0, \quad t = 0,$$

and when

$$x = 1, \quad t = \tfrac{1}{2}\pi.$$

(b) Integration by parts.

$$\int uv \, dx = u \int v \, dx - \int \left\{ \frac{du}{dx} \int v \, dx \right\} dx.$$

This is useful when one has to integrate the product of two functions, one of which (v) does not get any nastier when integrated, and the other of which (u) gets nicer when differentiated. For example, v may be an exponential or circular function, and u a power of x. For example

$$\int x \, e^x \, dx = x \, e^x - \int e^x \, dx = e^x(x-1).$$

(c) General advice.

Practice.

Look it up in a table of standard integrals.

Most functions can't be integrated, but you can always plot a graph and count up the squares.

SUGGESTIONS FOR FURTHER READING

This book is not intended to be a substitute for an elementary text-book on the calculus. It could be used in conjunction with such a text—for example:

Maxwell, E. A. (1954). *An Analytical Calculus*. Cambridge University Press. Four volumes, of which the first presents the basic ideas with greater rigour and coherence than I have attempted.

If you are interested in seeing how the ideas in this book can be developed further, the following books will show you. In some cases, they require more mathematical knowledge than is assumed in the present book; I have indicated where this is the case.

Goodwin, B. C. (1963). *Temporal Organisation in Cells*. Academic Press: New York. A first attempt to develop a dynamic theory of cellular control processes. The second half of the book requires further mathematics.

Grodins, F. S. (1963). *Control Theory and Biological Systems*. Columbia University Press: New York. An account of the mathematics used in control theory, and of their application in respiratory and cardiovascular physiology.

Haldane, J. B. S. (1932). *The Causes of Evolution*. Longmans, Green and Co., London. One of the books which established modern evolution theory. The appendices provide an introduction to the mathematical theory of evolution.

Li, C. C. (1955). *Population Genetics*. University of Chicago Press. A general account in which the mathematical treatment has been kept as simple as possible.

Lotka, A. J. (1956). *Elements of Mathematical Biology*. Dover Publications: New York. A classic, first published in 1924. Still an excellent source of ideas. Only occasionally demands additional mathematics.

Slobodkin, L. B. (1961). *Growth and Regulation of Animal Populations*. Holt, Rinehart and Winston, New York. The approach throughout is quantitative, but mathematics has been kept to the minimum.

Waterman, T. H. & Morowitz, H. J. (eds). (1965). *Theoretical and Mathematical Biology*. Blaisdell Publishing Company: New York. A collection of articles covering a wide range of topics.

ANSWERS TO EXAMPLES

Chapter 1

1 Concentration gradient $\propto L^{-1}$, and hence $P \propto L$.

2 $V \propto P^{0.5}$.

3 Food and water consumed at a rate $\propto L^2$, and hence distance $\propto L$.

4 Power required to fly $\propto L^{3.5} g^{1.5} \rho^{-0.5}$ and hence

$$W \simeq 59 \times 2/3 = 39 \cdot 3 \text{ lb wt. locally:}$$

for constant speed and size, $1 + j \propto g^{-1}$, and hence greyhound spends $2/3$ of time off ground.

5 At first sight, if cilia cover surface, power developed by cilia $\propto L^2$, and so power available should increase as rapidly as power required. But there is no point in a cilium lashing at water which has already been set moving by its neighbours.

Chapter 2

1 (a) $C < -\frac{1}{2}$; (b) $-\frac{1}{2} < C < 0$; (c) $0 < C < 1$; (d) $C > 1$.

2 $y_n = 2^{1-n/2} \sin n\pi/4$, $y_{10} = 1/16$.

3 (a) $X_E = 20$, $Y_E = 3$; (b) $y_{n+2} - 2y_{n+1} + 2y_n = 0$.

(c) An oscillation of increasing amplitude.

(d) Not at all.

(e) If the density of a prey and a predator are each limited only by the other, and if generations are separate, oscillations of large amplitude will ensue.

Chapter 3

1 (a) 60 mins;   (b) 54 mins.

2 (a) $4 \cdot 17 \times 10^8$ cells/ml.;   (b) $5 \cdot 13 \times 10^8$ cells/ml.

3   182·1 mins.

4 (*a*) 245;   (*b*) 247·5;   (*c*) 495;   (*d*) 120.

Chapter 4

1 (*a*) 1/9;   (*b*) 2/9;   (*c*) 5/6.

2 (*a*) 1/6;   (*b*) $\frac{2}{3}$;   (*c*) 3/10.

3 (*a*) 0·00198;   (*b*) 1·85 × 10^{-5}.

4 (*a*) 27/64;   (*b*) 175/256;   (*c*) 3/16;   (*d*) 0·0264.

5   3/16.

6 (*a*) 31/48;   (*b*) 1/17.

7   No.

Chapter 5

2 Yes.   **3** 50246.   **4** 1/19.   **6** 1/16;

  (*a*) 2·5 × 10^{-5};   (*b*) 3·36 × 10^{-4}.

7 $1 + (I_0 - 1)/2^n$.

Chapter 6

1 No; 419.   **2** 102.   **3** 11.   **4** $P = 1 - e^{-kt^2}$.

Chapter 7

1 $x = e^{-\pi/\sqrt{2}} \simeq 0.22$, when $t = \pi/\sqrt{2} \simeq 2\cdot22$.

2 (*a*) i, 2530; ii, 1495; (*b*) 0·098 sec.; 0·059 sec.; (*c*) 2·9°.

3 $dx_A/dt = kA - [k + K(B - A)] x_A - Kx_A^2$.

5 Anticlockwise spirals of decreasing radius about the origin.

INDEX

acceleration, work done in, 11, 12, 15
activation energy, of molecules, 105–7
age structure of populations, 39, 50–5
ageing, Szilard's theory of, 3, 87, 97
air
 viscous effects in small-scale flow of, 14
 work done in overcoming resistance of, 11–12
Argand diagram, 133

bacteria
 bacteriophage infection of, 90–2, 94–5
 logarithmic growth of, 40
bacteriophages, target theory and, 89, 90–2, 94–5
Bayes' theorem, 68, 70
bending stresses, ability to withstand, 7–8
binary fission, populations reproducing by, 39, 40
binomial expansion, 139
binomial theorem, 59–61, 93
blood
 count of cells in, 95
 rate of flow of, 9–10
blood groups, 66–9, 72, 85
Boltzmann's principle, 106
bone, ability to withstand stresses in, 7–8

centre of gravity, work done in raising, 11, 15
chemical reactions
 diffusion and, 123–6
 kinetics of, 105–7
chromosomes, damage to, 88, 93
cilia, movement by, 17
circular functions, 130–1
competition between species, 46–50
complex numbers, 131–4

compression, ability to withstand, 7
computer, occasions for calculation by, 2, 5, 43, 113, 126
cubes, length, surface area, and volume of, 6–7

delayed regulation of populations, 23–5, 54, 105, 113
differential equations
 to describe continuous-breeding populations, 39
 linear, 136–8
 partial, 117–19, 126
 reduction of, to linear form, 139–40
 replacement of recurrence relations by, 74
differentiation, 140–1
diffusion, 119–22
 rate of, across a surface, 16, 119
 and simultaneous chemical reaction, 123–6
diving, duration of, 12–13

ecology, application of Poisson series to, 95–6
efficiency, of conversion of chemical into mechanical energy by muscles, 9
energy
 of activation of molecules, 105–7
 muscular, 9
enzymes
 and activation energy, 106, 107
 in control of protein synthesis, 108–13
epidemics, 126
equations
 choice of appropriate, 2
 numerical methods of solving, 4–5, 41–3, 51–2
 see also differential equations, finite difference equations

standing wave, development of, 124–5
statistics, 1, 66
surface
  area of, and size, 7
  diffusion across, 16, 119
  loss of heat through, 9

target theory, 87–96
temperature
  and equilibrium of reaction, 107
  and rate of reaction, 106, 107
tensile strength, of muscles and tendons, 10
tension, ability to withstand, 7
twins, monovular and binovular, 66–8, 69

variables
  dependent and independent, 117
  elimination of, from equations, 29, 31, 37, 112

velocity
  and air resistance, 11–12
  force varying with, in control of muscle movement, 100–1
  and 'jumpiness' of gait, 16
  of running, and size of animal, 10, 12
viruses, target theory and, 89, 90–2, 94–5
viscosity
  effects from, in small-scale flow of air, 14
  of muscle, resistance to motion by, 100, 101, 103, 104
volume, and size, 7

weight
  maximum, for flying animals, 14
  proportional to volume, 7
wheels, advantage of, 11
work, done by muscles, 10–15